EDU

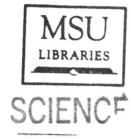

Clinical Training
and
Health Care Costs

Clinical Training
and
Health Care Costs:
A Basic Curriculum
for Medical Education

Mohan L. Garg, Sc.D.
Professor, Health Professions Education
Center for Educational Development
University of Illinois

and

Warren M. Kleinberg, M.D., M.P.H.
Director
Pediatric Ambulatory Services
St. Vincent Medical Center

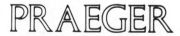

PRAEGER SPECIAL STUDIES • PRAEGER SCIENTIFIC

New York • Philadelphia • Eastbourne, UK
Toronto • Hong Kong • Tokyo • Sydney

Library of Congress Cataloging in Publication Data

Garg, Mohan L., 1933–
    Clinical training and health care costs.

    Bibliography: p.
    Includes index.
    1. Medical care—United States—Cost control—
Study and teaching.   2. Medicine—Study and teaching—
United States.   I. Kleinberg, Warren M., 1944–
II. Title.   [DNLM: 1. Cost Control.   2. Curriculum.
3. Education, Medical.   4. Health Services—economics.
W 18 G231c]
RA410.53.G37   1984   610′.68′1   84-15152
ISBN 0-03-069882-0

Published in 1985 by Praeger Publishers
CBS Educational and Professional Publishing
A Division of CBS, Inc.
521 Fifth Avenue, New York, New York 10175 U.S.A.

© 1984 by Praeger Publishers

456789   145   987654321

Printed in the United States of America

Contents

To our wives for support
and encouragement
To our children whose future we
hope to sustain

Foreword

Nothing is more gratifying than watching seeds sprout and grow into sturdy plants. Hence it is a pleasure to write a foreword to a book which represents the flowering of a seed planted by the National Fund for Medical Education in 1975. At that time, the idea that the cost of medical care might be contained in part through the education of the next generation of doctors had occurred to a few faculty members at the Medical College of Ohio at Toledo, but the vast majority of medical educators seemed blissfully unaware that the cost of medical care was even a problem. Among the few who might have been aware, there was no sense that the economic consequences of clinical decisions should figure in what medical students were taught. Thus when the Toledo group turned to the Fund to support a teaching experiment they had been developing for two years, they had no idea of the revolution they were starting in American medical education. Nor did the Fund. Those who approved the grant thought it was a high risk, yet this was consistent with the guiding philosophy of NFME's Innovative Grants Program—that an occasional seed might fall on fertile soil.

In the few years since the Toledo experiment began, the cost of medical care has become a major political issue, an overriding concern of American industry, and a threat to the future independence of doctors and hospitals. The importance of including "cost containment" in clinical teaching is now recognized by many educators, and most medical schools address the topic in some fashion. Experiments with various ways of teaching students how to make prudent use of clinical resources are now widespread. Further breakthroughs in educational techniques are to be expected, yet medical schools have an obligation to their current students. Educators need a sourcebook of tried and proven methods and materials for teaching how to conserve medical resources. That is the purpose of this book. It presents methods and materials in convenient modules which teachers can adapt to their own styles and circumstances.

Although some specifics of instruction will someday become obsolete, I think the Toledo curriculum has several attributes which will prove durable. First and foremost, it is *clinically oriented*; almost all teaching exercises are based on actual case records. Second, it is integrated into the curriculum from matriculation to graduation yet adds relatively few hours and readings. Third, cost and quality of care are always considered in parallel, as they must be if cost containment is not to become detrimental to patients' health. Finally, a variety of techniques—from conventional lectures to imaginative role-playing—are used.

The authors emphasize the key place of faculty, both as instructors and role models, in awakening students to the limits on the nation's wealth and in teaching them how to use resources prudently. Faculty commitment is prerequisite to the success of this new departure in medical education. The most carefully planned teaching exercises will have no lasting effect on the practice behavior of new physicians if the minds of clinical teachers remain closed to change. The director of a cost-containment project at another school epitomized the problem: "My faculty gives a student who wastes money on inappropriate tests and hospitalization a slap on the wrist; but missing the most unlikely possibility in a differential diagnosis is regarded as a mortal sin." Thus the students at that school score high on examinations on how to contain costs, but they are profligate in actual practice.

We, today's teachers, graduated into a world of burgeoning technology and seemingly limitless resources—a fool's paradise, we can see in retrospect, in which cost was no object and "quality of care" became corrupted to mean "do everything." Thus we face a tougher prospect than our students. Students' minds are open, and they can learn to include considerations of cost and benefit in clinical decisions as naturally as they do pathophysiology. This has been proven conclusively at Toledo. But our minds are burdened by habits and attitudes ingrained in a bygone era. This book will show you how to teach students; but if you let it, it will teach you too.

John Gordon Freymann, M.D., President
National Fund for Medical Education
Hartford, Connecticut

Preface

The Social Security Amendments of 1965 (PL 89-97) established the Medicare program to provide health services to the elderly. Under the retrospective payment system established for Medicare recipients, the health care system, including medical education, grew at a rapid rate and so did costs. Medicare expenditures increased from $3 billion in 1965 to $33 billion in 1982. From 1979 to 1982 the average cost of a hospital day increased almost 18 percent a year. During this period of growth, the education of physicians was influenced by the reimbursement policy. In teaching hospitals, the patient expected to receive the most up-to-date treatment. The resident not only ordered whatever was appropriate for the patient but also what would further his or her own education. The faculty actively, or by default, encouraged the resident's behavior. Teaching hospitals became institutions where the most modern technology and the newest tests and procedures were employed. This standard of practice influenced undergraduate, graduate and continuing medical education. It is not surprising, therefore, that the costs of treating patients in teaching hospitals exceeded those in all other types of hospitals.

However, Congress enacted PL 98-21 in 1983, which, by creation of the Prospective Payment System (PPS), completely restructures the

Medicare reimbursement of hospital inpatient services. For this purpose, the Health Care Financing Administration (HCFA) has developed 467 categories called "Diagnosis Related Groups" (DRGs) of which 356 are presently applicable to Medicare patients. Formulas have been developed by HCFA to estimate the cost of each DRG with proper consideration for the size of the hospital, severity of cases, and other factors. Appropriate consideration was also given to incorporating the costs of graduate medical education, and capital expenditures. Thus, under PPS there will be an upper reimbursable limit for each DRG. The government will no longer be specifically concerned with length of stay (LOS) or numbers of laboratory tests and procedures and their costs.

This sweeping regulation will require close cooperation between hospital administrators and physicians. In order to stay within DRG limits, physicians will have to develop mechanisms to control the two most important contributors to costly inpatient services, the length of stay and ancillary services. This will inevitably lead to a reexamination of a whole set of issues related to quality assurance and cost containment.

To control escalating costs, the federal government legislated Professional Standards Review Organizations (PSROs) in 1972. These groups emphasized a review mechanism based upon LOS for Medicare/Medicaid patients. Since then, LOS review has been the primary criterion against which most hospital cost-control activities have been carried out.

However, length of stay is only one contributing factor to hospital costs. Although average lengths of stay have been decreasing, total costs are still rising. In today's health-care system it is possible to generate quickly costs of several thousand dollars for individual patients by utilizing high technology services such as C.T. scans, cardiac catheterization, and radio-nucleide studies. Also, low-cost items such as blood chemistries, when added together, may contribute significantly to total expenditures.

Despite the enormous growth of diagnostic tests and procedures, the main criterion to determine appropriateness of hospital treatment still revolves around LOS. Even the DRGs were created using LOS as a primary contributing variable. However, a cost/benefit study conducted by HCFA in 1979 determined that PSROs were marginally effective. A preliminary study by the authors suggests that a review mechanism based solely on LOS does not include significant cost-generating activities. The main findings of this research were:

1. The charges for diagnostic tests, procedures and therapy generated by physicians accumulate very rapidly (50 percent by the end of the fifth day of hospitalization and 75 percent by the end of the ninth day).

2. The rate of accumulation is similar irrespective of diagnosis, its complexities, or type of insurance.

The above results suggest that the *LOS review alone may not provide the basis for an efffective approach to control of hospital costs.* In 1982, $136 billion was spent on hospital care. Nearly 40 percent, or $54.4 billion, was spent on ancillary services and 60 percent or $81.6 billion went for room and board. Assuming that the rate of accumulation derived from the sample is nationally applicable, $27.2 billion for ancillary services is accumulated by the end of the fourth day and $40.8 billion by the end of the eighth day. *Therefore, any review system that begins after the eighth day of stay would affect only $13.6 billion; $40.8 billion of expenditures for ancillary services would never be reviewed.*

The advent of the new reimbursement system requires that new approaches to physicians' education be developed to limit rising costs. And to be effective, the educational approaches should include LOS review but shift their emphasis to ancillary services. The educational emphasis presented in the books, therefore, primarily revolves around diagnostic tests, procedures, and therapies ordered by the physician. The impression made upon medical students during their clinical training is carried over into their medical practices. Each part of the cost-containment curriculum presented in this book is a complete unit that can be integrated with others and implemented in many medical school programs. Moreover, some of the parts, even though primarily developed for undergraduate medical education during clinical years, can be readily applied in graduate and continuing medical education. For example, to cut costs of inpatient care, several medical societies and the American Hospital Association have encouraged utilization of preadmission testing.

In short, the curriculum presented here revolves around the process level of the medical care system (what the physicians do for their patients), during which attitudes and behaviors are formed. The adoption of parts of the curriculum developed and presented here will, therefore, add another dimension to medical education with respect to the cost and the benefit of each action taken by physicians for their patients.

MLG
WMK

Acknowledgments

We owe a debt of gratitude to Dr. Jack Mulligan whose foresight helped establish and develop the initial student education program. We are also grateful for the assistance of Mr. Werner Gliebe in developing the resident and practicing physician cost-awareness programs and in reviewing the drafts for this book. We wish to thank all the physicians, directors of medical education, and faculty who participated and facilitated the cost-awareness education programs, and give special recognition to Dr. Larry Frenkel, Dr. Mounir ElKhatib, Dr. Ramon Rodriguez-Torres, Dr. Paul Baehren, Dr. Ed Pike, and Dr. Howard Madigan. We enjoyed the support and cooperation of the administration and faculty of the Medical College of Ohio at Toledo, and the Presidents of the Ohio State Medical Association, Drs. C. Douglass Ford and Baird Pfahl. Not least of all was the enthusiasm and support of the medical students, residents, and practicing physicians of Northwest Ohio.

1 Introduction: The Need for an Educational Program in Cost Containment for Future Physicians

The physician's position in society, the task assigned to him and the rules of conduct imposed upon him changed in every period. They were determined primarily by the social and economic structure of society and by the technical and scientific means available to medicine at the time.

—Henry Sigerist
Medicine and Human Welfare

If physicians are to continue to have an effective voice in our own affairs, a new dimension must be added. Physicians must be as concerned about the cost of medical care as they have traditionally been concerned with its quality.

—George Dunlop, President
American College of Surgeons

Physicians influence, if not control, almost 70 percent of all expenditures for health care by their decisions. From 1965 to 1981 health care expenditures in the United States increased from $41.7 billion to $286.6 billion. In 1981, health care costs increased 15.1 percent on top of a 15.8 percent rise in 1980. Medical costs currently absorb 9.8 percent of the Gross National Product. With their large impact on health care costs, physicians can play a significant role in reducing those costs.

The way physicians practice medicine throughout their careers is influenced by the knowledge, skills, and attitudes acquired through educational experiences. Their knowledge determines which patients go into the hospital, how long they stay, what diagnostic and treatment services they receive, and what prescriptions they will take as outpatients. Some studies have suggested that increased emphasis on training future physicians in cost containment techniques can produce lower costs (Report of the Government Accounting Office [G.A.O.] 1982).

The traditional views of their profession held by most physicians leave them ill-equipped to deal with cost issues. Henry Sigerist observed in his book, *Medicine and Human Welfare:*

> trained as highly specialized scientists, [physicians] are unprepared to grapple with problems that are primarily social and economic. They have built for themselves a legendary, sentimental, and romantic history of their profession, to which they cling desperately, and which determines their actions.

As the role of physicians has become even more complex, owing to factors such as specialization and improved technology, the consequences of their decisions have multiplied. They include obligating patients, public agencies and other third-party payers to increasing expenses.

If physicians influence directly about 70 percent of this nation's burgeoning medical costs, few of them have been prepared by their educations for their "executive" responsibilities as directors of the health-care team.

> At the beginning of the century [when most relationships were simple doctor-patient] two out of every three persons employed in the health field were physicians; today, the proportion is one of every 12. (Fuchs, 1979)

A major reason for cost-control pressures is the soaring government role in reimbursements. The percentage of payments for health services that comes out of consumers' pockets—directly and through private medical insurance—has declined, while the ratio of payment for health care from public funds has almost doubled (Figure 1.1 and Table 1.1). In 1965, Americans paid directly 17 percent of the health care funds that went to hospitals, and their insurers paid 42 percent; 39 percent was paid to hospitals by governmental agencies and 2 percent by other sources. By 1981, only 11 percent of hospital costs was paid directly by consumers, and 33 percent by their insurers. However, 54 percent was paid to hospitals through government reimbursements (Figure 1.2).

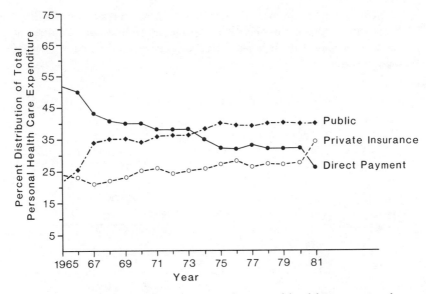

FIGURE 1.1. Percent distribution of personal health-care expenditures.

The same trend is evident in payments to physicians. Consumers paid directly 61 percent of the money that went to physicians in 1965, and their insurer paid 32 percent; governmental agencies paid only 7 percent. Just 16 years later, in 1981, consumers paid directly 38 percent of physicians' fees, and their insurers paid a similar 35 percent. With the onset of Medicaid and Medicare in 1965, payments through local, state and federal governments grew to 27 percent (Figure 1.3).

The shift to payments from the public sector—along with the burgeoning costs—has created political pressures to make the medical profession accountable. The Secretary of Health, Education and Welfare reminded the 1978 annual meeting of the Association of American Medical Colleges that health care had become the nation's third-largest industry, and added:

> medical schools must take a more active role in making physicians responsive to demographic, social and economic changes which have deep implications for health care.... The medical education system can do more to train physicians to be attentive to the expense they generate, as well as the services they provide and order up.
>
> ...[W]e must face the enormous implications of runaway health care costs. We are approaching the day, in health care, as in the field

of energy, when we simply cannot sustain the costs of chrome-finned, gas-guzzling, option-rich technology. Medical technology certainly has its uses. But it must be applied judiciously on a strong science base. (Califano, 1979)

An economist told the same meeting:

The elimination of unnecessary surgery, hospital admissions, tests, prescriptions, and the like is the surest, swiftest, safest way of stopping the runaway inflation of health care costs. (Fuchs, 1979)

TABLE 1.1. National Expenditures for Hospital and Physician Services by Source of Funds for Selected Years

	Year			
Type/Source	1981	1975	1970	1965
	Billions of Dollars			
Hospitals	$118.0 (100)*	$52.1 (100)	$27.8 (100)	$13.9 (100)
Consumer	52.2 (44)	22.7 (44)	12.8 (46)	8.2 (59)
Direct	12.8 (11)	4.3 (8)	2.8 (10)	2.4 (17)
Insurance	39.4 (33)	18.4 (36)	10.0 (36)	5.8 (42)
Public	64.1 (54)	28.8 (55)	14.6 (53)	5.4 (39)
Federal	48.7 (41)	20.3 (39)	9.4 (34)	2.4 (18)
State & Local	15.4 (13)	8.6 (16)	5.2 (19)	3.0 (21)
Other	1.7 (1)	0.5	0.4 (1)	0.3 (2)
Physician Services	54.8 (100)	29.9 (100)	14.3 (11)	8.5 (100)
Consumer	39.8 (73)	18.4 (74)	11.2 (78)	7.9 (93)
Direct	20.8 (38)	8.7 (35)	6.3 (44)	5.2 (61)
Insurance	19.0 (35)	9.7 (39)	4.9 (34)	2.7 (32)
Public	15.0 (27)	6.5 (26)	3.1 (22)	0.6 (7)
Federal	11.6 (21)	4.7 (19)	2.2 (16)	0.2 (2)
State & Local	3.3 (6)	1.9 (7)	0.9 (6)	0.4 (5)
Other	—	0.1	—	—

*Indicates column percent.

Source: Gibson, Robert M., and Daniel R. Waldo: "National Health Expenditures, 1981." Health Care Finance Review 4:1 (September 1981): 1–35.

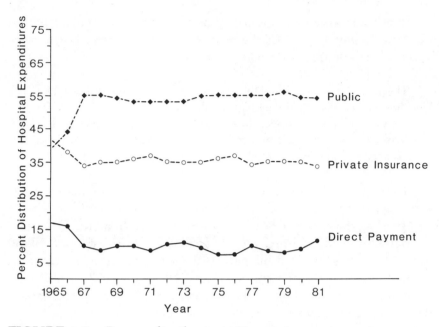

FIGURE 1.2. Percent distribution of hospital expenditures by source of funds since 1965.

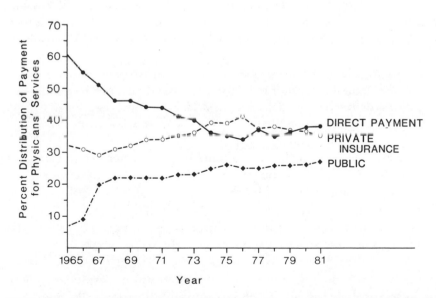

FIGURE 1.3. Percent distribution of payment for physicians' services by source of funds since 1965.

Physicians have been described as "gatekeepers" (Fuchs, 1974) and "purchasing agents" of the vast health-care system, but a more down-to-earth image is offered by one writer:

> The physician may be thought of as a shopper in a grocery store. The shopping cart is like the patient, being loaded with items from the shelves. The smart shopper, like a good physician, decides whether to place an item on the cart, based on his knowledge of the cost and his need of it. (Dresnick et al., 1979)

The supermarket image may be less dignified, but it is just as apt. A knowledge of costs is a vital qualification for today's physician, who is both steering the complex health care system and "loading the cart."

But how well qualified are physicians to deal with controlling costs? "The physician and his patient are usually not even cognizant of the costs of basic hospital services" (Redisch, 1978), although almost 40 percent of all medical care costs are attributable to hospital service charges. Physicians generally use hospitals inefficiently for three reasons:

1. They do not perceive the cost of hospital care, because their services and those of the hospital are billed separately. Physicians frequently turn over many of their duties to other hospital professionals but continue to bill patients as if they had provided the care themselves.

> Examples of this trend include the obstetrician who relies more and more on the nursing staff and who rushes in at the last minute for the actual delivery, or the attending physician who utilizes house staff to care for his patients on Wednesdays and Saturdays. (Redisch, 1978)

Instead of charging less to patients because other health care professionals provide a portion of care, physicians usually continue to charge the same fees. Aided by the separation of bills for the costs of joint hospital-and-physician services, the physician has shown a great willingness to bill as much in his "supervisory" capacity over hospital inputs as when he performs services directly.

2. Physicians do not know the cost of routine hospital services, because hospitals prorate the charges among all patients. Because they are unaware of the costs of such services, physicians tend to make too much use of them.

3. Physicians' attitudes about hospitalizing patients are influenced by their awareness that a third party—not the patient—will pay.

> To the extent that hospital care is more heavily insured than ambulatory physician care, the physician is likely to suggest a hospital stay for a patient who could be treated as well [and more efficiently] on an ambulatory basis. (Redisch, 1978)

Another factor is that:

> it is the physician who typically engages in a lobbying effort with hopes of committing the [hospital] administrator and trustees to invest in additional bed space, in personnel to help him provide more and better patient care, and in new and expensive technology. (Redisch, 1978)

Indeed, the proliferation of new technology was recently called by Fuchs the most powerful long-term explanation for rising costs.

Overuse and misuse of laboratory tests also cause major cost problems. One study (Griner and Liptzin, 1971) indicated that more than one-fourth of the average patient's hospital bills consisted of laboratory charges. This study also indicated that, from 1965 to 1970, the percentage of increase in laboratory costs was more than double the increase in overall hospital costs. The researchers concluded that the greater use of diagnostic tests had ultimately led to their overuse and that, although this may not necessarily be harmful to a patient's health, it certainly is harmful to the pocketbooks of those who pay for hospital care. Several studies also reported that large numbers of a medical school's clinical faculty, house staffs, and students most consistently underestimated the costs of tests (Roth, 1973; Skipper et al., 1975, 1976; Robertson, 1980).

A similar but broader-based study included more than 350 faculty members and house staffers at a major center. Only 46 percent of any of the sample groups estimated test costs "correctly," even though answers were counted as "correct" if they varied no more than 10 percent in either direction from the actual cost. Underestimates were prevalent. The researchers concluded:

> Cost awareness should be included in medical school curricula and residency programs. Teaching institutions have an obligation to teach not only the latest in medical knowledge, but also to teach the

indications for tests and procedures with consideration of risks, benefits and costs.... (Dresnick et al., 1979)

Besides the fact that many physicians do not know how much tests cost, the proliferation of tests seems, inevitably, to lead to increased use. A physician could order from among fewer than 100 laboratory tests in 1950; in 1980, from more than 600. For patients with myocardial infarction, physicians who were included in one study took an average of one X ray and five electrocardiograms in 1964; in 1971, the average for the same medical problem was six X rays and nine electrocardiograms. Increased use of diagnostic tests does not, however, necessarily mean better care for patients, though it does greatly affect costs.

> What seems remarkably clear is that medical students receive precious little information or experience that would permit them to become knowledgeable in evaluating, on a scientific basis, the outcome of medical intervention. [Yet] a thorough grounding in the process of evaluation research might well enhance the efficiency of physician decision-making. (Carrol and Becker, 1975)

One of the most obvious opportunities for helping physicians control costs is the inclusion of cost containment as a part of medical education. Yet few medical schools offer such instruction, and little is available as continuing education programs for physicians already in practice. Some critics and leaders of the medical establishment agree that since physicians dominate the cost structure, changing physicians' behavior by education seems to be the most effective tool for attacking the problem of increasing costs.

The president of the American College of Surgeons (Dunlop, 1976) told his group:

> Industry and government are now paying our bills and, like it or not, we must be able to answer their questions, project our future, defend the positions we take, and have data to support our contentions....
>
> We should look twice at our day-to-day practice habits. The extra chest plate or blood gas sample, or the extra half-day of hospitalization may be popular "defensive medicine," but are they always necessary? Multiplied, they can be a greater burden to the financing system than, perhaps, any other single factor.

An editorial in the *Journal of Medical Education* (McGinnis, 1976), entitled "The Rising Costs of Hospital Care: Mandate for Academic Introspection," stated:

> Medical school and house staff training programs should intensify their efforts to incorporate consideration of costs into hospital practice....
>
> [T]he recent and disturbing increase in hospital costs cannot be blamed only on inflation or inept administrative policies. Rather, the principal share of the responsibility lies in the physician practices and the available technology—both of which can be considerably influenced by the programs of academic training centers....

Better clinical decision-making, which will save money and minimize patient risk, is effected by governmental and public pressures. Such decision-making is totally consistent with high quality medical care. Medical educators must create programs incorporating information on the economics of health care, the causes of rising health-care costs, and the physicians's role in controlling these costs. Effective programs must make changes in physicians' behavior part of their medical practice.

It is with these concerns in mind that this study is being made available. The authors initiated cost-containment instruction at the Medical College of Ohio, Toledo, in 1973. It was one of the nation's first efforts to integrate such instruction into a medical school curriculum.

This work is intended as a sourcebook for medical schools, hospitals and professional organizations, so that educational strategies already developed can be used without being reinvented. The advantages, disadvantages and resource commitments required for each educational strategy — or module—and the extent to which a module might best be presented, singly or in combination with others, are considered, so that the program planner can select the means most appropriate to his or her own educational context. A clinical faculty committed to support and reinforce training in cost-effective decision making will make the difference between a successful program and a token effort.

REFERENCES

1.   Califano, J.A., Jr. "The Government Medical Education Partnership." *Journal of Medical Education* 54:1 (January 1979): 19–26.

2. Carrol, J., and Becker, S. "The Paucity of Course Work in Medical Care Evaluation." *Journal of Medical Education* 50:1 (1975): 31–37.

3. Dunlop, G.R. "Medical Costs—Our Common Dilemma." *American College of Surgeons Bulletin* (November 1976): 7–11.

4. Dresnick, S.J., et al. "The Physician's Role in the Cost-Containment Problem." *JAMA* 241:15 (1979): 1606–1609.

5. Fuchs, V.R. *Who Shall Live? Health Economics and Social Choice* (New York: Basic Books, 1974).

6. ———. "Public Policy and the Medical Establishment." *Journal of Medical Education* 54 (1979): 8–11.

7. The U.S. General Accounting Office, Washington, D.C. *Physician Cost-Containment Training Can Reduce Medical Costs*, HRD-82-36 (February 4, 1982).

8. Gibson, R.M., and Waldo, D.R. "National Health Expenditures, 1981." *Health Care Finance Review* 4:1 (September 1981): 1–35.

9. Griner, P., and Liptzin, B. "Use of the Laboratory in a Teaching Hospital." *Annals of Internal Medicine* 75 (1971): 157–163.

10. McGinnis, J.M. "The Rising Costs of Hospital Care: Mandate for Academic Introspection." Editorial: *Journal of Medical Education* 51 (1976): 602–604.

11. Redisch, M.A. "Physician Involvement in Hospital Decision Making 1978." In *Hospital Cost Containment—Selected Notes for Future Policy*. Edited by M. Zubkoff, Raskin, I.E., and Hanft, R.S. (New York: Prodist, 1978), pp. 217–243.

12. Robertson, W.D. "Costs of Diagnostic Tests: Estimates by Health Professionals." *Medical Care* 18:5 (1980): 556–559.

13. Roth, R. "How Do We Spend Your Patients' Dollars?" *Prison* 1 (September 1973): 16–18.

14. Skipper, J.K., Smith, G., Mulligan, J.L., and Garg, M.L. "Medical Students' Unfamiliarity with the Cost of Diagnostic Tests." *Journal of Medical Education* 50 (1975): 683–684.

15. Skipper, J.K., Smith, G., Mulligan, J.L. and Garg, M.L. "Physicians' Knowledge of Cost: The Case of Diagnostic Tests." *Inquiry* 13 (1976): 194–198.

2   Cost Containment: An Overview of the Instructional Program at the Medical College of Ohio

A belief in the 'technologic imperative' prevails; physicians are much more concerned with providing as much treatment as possible with using the most modern equipment and techniques than they are with managing health care resources efficiently.
—National Association of Blue Cross Plans, 1977

The Medical College of Ohio at Toledo initiated a program in 1973 to develop and implement a curriculum in quality assurance and cost containment. The following goals were set for the undergraduate students:

    1. To familiarize the students with the costs of medical care and the role of the physician as a "generator of costs" and "captain of the team."

    2. To study national trends and legislation on quality assurance and cost containment.

    3. To consider methods of evaluating the three components of the medical care system: structure, process, and outcome.

    4. To introduce the legal implications of various national quality assurance programs.

Initial experience of the program convinced the originators that the key to the success of any effort lies in making it clinically oriented. "Students want to learn medicine; they will learn other concepts, as long as the medical ones are not ignored" (Garg et al., 1980). Moreover, it became apparent that it is important to gain as much clinical faculty

11

support and participation as possible in order to guarantee that such concepts become an integral and legitimate part of the medical socialization process. In other words, students must know that both the faculty and their peers believe it is desirable to be a cost-conscious practicing physician.

Rather than "add on" another course, the cost-containment curriculum at the Medical College of Ohio was integrated into existing medical school courses so as to require minimal additional contact hours. An attempt was made to teach medical students to recognize and seek out alternatives to costly medical care, while at the same time not compromising the quality of the care delivered. The students were taught to weigh alternatives carefully from the standpoint of empirical and tested medical knowledge.

After preliminary attempts to provide a cost-containment curriculum, it became clear that, to be a success, instruction in cost containment must be flexible and adapted to different educational environments. The program was integrated into the Medical College's three year multidisciplinary integrated curriculum. The three year curriculum consisted of:

Phase I. Biological Concepts of Disease: Lasting about 14 weeks, it was designed to present the human and cellular biology essential to understanding disease.

Phase II. Basic Science and Clinical Aspects of Each of the Ten Organ Systems: Running for about 18 months, it consisted of hematology, oncology, and immunology; the cardiovascular system; the respiratory system; the digestive system; the endocrine system; the reproductive system; the urinary system; the nervous system and behavior; the locomotor system; and infectious diseases.

Phase III. Clinical Clerkships: It consisted of 11 months of clerkships, and emphasized development of clinical and patient management skills through a team approach working towards health maintenance. The clerkships were expanded to 14 months in 1977.

The Cost-Containment Curriculum was integrated in the following manner:

Phase I. Biological Concepts of Disease: The teaching in Phase I consisted of 90 minutes of lecture time covering such topics as the

Social Security Act of 1965, which created the Medicare and Medicaid reimbursement programs; the Professional Standards Review Organization (PRSO) legislation of 1972, intended to assure quality and contain costs; and the ramifications of peer review for the future practice of medicine. Students were also introduced to the three levels of evaluation of medical care: structure, process, and outcomes. A brief review of assessment techniques was presented including structural evaluations, such as the accreditation requirements, the Joint Commission on Accreditation of Hospitals, the effects of the Flexner Report on quality of undergraduate medical education, and recent developments in board certification and subspecialty training requirements. The main goals were to expose students to the history of quality assurance techniques, to various reimbursement mechanisms for health care, and to social and public presures for control of quality and cost.

Phase II. The Ten Organ Systems: Teaching was begun during Phase II through presentation of one clinical pathological conference (CPC) in each of four selected body systems. The selection was made to spread the curriculum evenly over the entire 18 months. The CPC uses the fundamental disciplines in medicine, and integrates them for clinical problem solving and education. To present cost awareness, a cost/benefit analysis of the diagnostic workup and treatment scheduled was added to the existing protocol and presentation.

Students were provided with case information for the CPC in three sections:

1. General description of the case, with descriptive and objective findings and assessment.
2. Patient progress summary for each day, divided into subjective and objective findings in assessment.
3. A day by day list of diagnostic test results ordered by the resident or the attending physician plus a treatment schedule. The cost of laboratory tests ordered was included on the laboratory flow sheet.

For the presentation of the CPC, five students were selected from the class. The first four presented traditional components of the CPC and the last student presented a cost/benefit analysis of the laboratory workup and treatment plan. The set of materials developed for the CPC and used successfully is shown in Figures 2.1, 2.2, 2.3, 2.4, and Table

FIGURE 2.1. Reprinted with permission from: Garg, M.L., Gliebe, W.A., Kleinberg, W.M.: "The Way We Teach Cost Containment," *Medical Teacher*, 2:5 (1980):222–228.

Introductory Session: Orientation Day

---

1. Define structure, process, and outcome in relation to evaluating the quality of medical care.
2. Review epidemiological concepts for determining health care.
3. Explain assignment for subsequent seminars.

6.1 of Chapter 6, in which a more detailed discussion of the CPC technique is provided.

Phase III. Clinical Clerkships: The curriculum during Phase III consisted of several experimental attempts that evolved over the years as the faculty gained experience. The curriculum was integrated into the Community Medicine and Ambulatory Care Clerkship. Initially, chart audits with emphasis solely on assessment of quality were stressed. Implicit and explicit criteria, and a combination of both, were utilized. However, as more knowledge was gained, the teaching strategies were modified. The concept of tracers (Kessner, et al., 1973a, 1973b) was introduced, following publication of the report by the Institute of Medicine. Important advantages of the tracer approach included the availability of management plans for six common medical conditions. The concept was made more powerful when later combined with disease staging as proposed by Gonnella and Goran (1976). The combination of tracers with staging provided the students with an intensive, in-depth exposure to quality decision-making concepts which related to outcome.

When the cost-containment curriculum was fully developed and implemented during this phase, it consisted of a one hour orientation session and three 90 minute seminars in each of the subsequent three weeks during the four week clinical clerkship. During orientation, students were given their assignments for chart audit and an outline for the subsequent seminars along with essential readings. Each student was given a complete chart of one patient with a selected medical problem of

FIGURE 2.2. Seminar 1. Quality assurance. Reprinted with permission from: Garg, M.L., Gliebe, W.A., Kleinberg, W.M.: "The Way We Teach Cost Containment," *Medical Teacher*, 2:5 (1980):222–228.

---

1. Each student reports on one of the topics below:

    (a) Discuss the strengths and limitations of the different methods of quality assessment.
    (b) Define the concept of tracer disease with its minimum care plan, the level of analysis for which it appears appropriate and its strengths and limitations.
    (c) Define the concept of staging for relating process to outcome.
    (d) Discuss whether quality of care can be improved using the above approaches.
    (e) Compare the findings of Nobrega et al. with that of Brook and Appel.

2. General discussion of alternative existing mechanisms of quality control.

    (a) Performance Evaluation Procedures for Auditing and Improving Patient Care (PEP) program of the Joint Commission on Hospital Accreditation.
    (b) Mandatory Continuing Medical Education for Licensure.
    (c) Specialty recertification.

Reading List

1. Brook, Robert H. and Appel, F.A., "Quality Care Assessment: Choosing a Method of Peer Review." *New England Journal of Medicine*, 288(1973):1323.
2. Kessner, David M., Kalk, C.K. and Singer, J., "Assessing Health Quality—The Case for Tracers." *New England Journal of Medicine*, 288(1973):189-194.
3. Gonnella, J.S., Louis, D.Z.. and McCord, J.J., "The Staging Concept—an Approach to Assessment of Outcome of Ambulatory Care," *Medical Care*, 14(1975):13-71
4. Nobrega, Fred T., et al., "Quality Assessment in Hypertension: Analysis of Process and Outcome Methods," *New England Journal of Medicine*, 296(1976):145-148.

---

the month. The problems selected were usually those listed as tracers: essential hypertension, middle ear infection and hearing loss, and urinary tract infection. These problems were selected because of their high frequency in hospital admissions and outpatient cases and the availability of explicit criteria for their management. The students were provided with manuals delineating all diagnostic tests and procedures and their charges in the hospital.

FIGURE 2.3. Seminar 2. Cost containment. (Medical Commons and Allocation of Scarce Resources). Reprinted with permission from: Garg, M.L., Gliebe, W.A., Kleinberg, W.M.: "The Way We Teach Cost Containment," *Medical Teacher*, 2:5 (1980):222–228.

---

1. Recommendations of National Commission on Cost of Medical Care:

   (a) Financing mechanisms (1-7).
   (b) Private sector cost containment initiatives (9-15).
   (c) Regulating mechanisms (16-25).
   (d) Medical practices to contain costs (26-32).
   (e) Educational efforts and cost containment (33-39; 46-48).
   (f) Defining quality; use of allied health personnel; cost assessment research (38, 40-45).

2. Government interventions as:

   (a) Educational tools.
   (b) Potentially punitive devices (such as proposed hospital cost increase ceiling).

Reading List

1. *National Commission on the Cost of Medical Care, Summary Report.* American Medical Association, Chicago, 1977.
2. Bennett Amendment (PL 92-603), *Appendix II.*
3. Jessee, W., Munier, W.B., Fielding, J., and Goran, M.J., PSRO: an educational force for improving quality of care, *New England Journal of Medicine*, 27 March 1975.
4. Reluctant MDs now face nonphysician PSROs, *Medical World News*, 16 May 1977.
5. A comparison of three approaches to medical care evaluation studies.
6. How doctors view hospital costs, *Medical World News*, 2 May 1977.
7. Hospital costs: biggest piece of the health care bill, *Medical World News*, 2 May 1977.
8. The AMA's health plan, *Medical World News*, 6 June 1977.
9. Can PSRO's control cost? *Journal of Legal Medicine*, May 1977.
10. Hiatt, H.H., Protecting the medical commons: who is responsible? *New England Journal of Medicine*, 1975, 293, 235-241.
11. Every meow of this cat costs $200, *Perspective*, Fall 1976.
12. Pinto, Richard S. and M.H. Becker, Computed tomography in paediatric diagnosis. *American Journal of Diseases of Childhood*, May 1977, 131.
13. Regulating physician's fees, *Medical World News*, 13 June 1977.
14. How doctors view regulation of their fees, *Medical World News*, 13 June 1977.

FIGURE 2.4. Seminar 3. Chart audit. Reprinted with permission from: Garg, M.L., Gliebe, W.A., Kleinberg, W.M.: "The Way We Teach Cost Containment," *Medical Teacher*, 2:5 (1980)222–228.

---

1. Each student reviews the chart of a hypertensive patient using implicit criteria for audit and reports in the form provided (see Chart Review below).

2. Discuss the chart audit process.

3. Discuss hypertension:
   (a) Tracer.
   (b) Staging.
   (c) Minimum care criteria.
   (d) Evaluation from a medical record.
   (e) Protocols versus compliance versus outcome.

4. Discuss hypertension:
   (a) PSRO criteria.
   (b) Hospitalization versus outpatient workup.

The three seminars are outlined in Figures 2.1, 2.2, 2.3, and 2.4 with appropriate assigned readings. Written assignments were also given and these assignments, along with the student's comments, constituted the basis for evaluation of the program.

In 1978, a reorganization of the clinical curriculum eliminated the one month clerkship in Community Medicine, and the time available was reduced to a one hour orientation and a three hour seminar during the pediatric clerkship. The faculty devised a new approach using selected national issues in health care costs. At that time the National Commission on the Cost of Medical Care (1977) published its recommendations for health care cost controls. While their recommendations were debated by the House of Delegates of the American Medical Association, the Carter Administration proposed a 9 percent ceiling on hospital cost increases to the Congress. The National Commission's report and the Administration's proposal were felt to be the key health care cost issues and were used as the basis for a new, modified curriculum in the limited time available.

A selected number of recommendations from the National Commission's report, bearing directly on the students' involvement during their four week pediatric rotations in the hospital, were chosen. At the orientation session, the students were given summaries of the National Commission's report and each group of two students was assigned two specific recommendations and asked to relate them to their own hospital experiences. During the last week of the rotation, a role-play workshop offered opportunities to "experience" various hospital planning dilemmas if the proposed 9 percent ceiling on hospital cost increases was enacted by the Congress. The workshop consisted of two parts. During the first part, the students discussed their reports on the earlier assigned National Commission recommendations. The second part consisted of a role-play workshop where each student played the part of a member of a hospital executive committee.

The role-play sessions were very successful from the standpoint of student participation, evaluation, and comments. Most students achieved the desired objectives for each seminar: to demonstrate the complexity of setting economic priorities and compromise solutions; to deal with limited resources and group problem solving. The students became keenly aware of the dilemmas of the influence of costs on the quality of medical care.

CONCLUSIONS

The cost-containment curriculum over the three curricular phases sought to present in a systematic way the broad economic, social, and political issues that influence the medical care process. By a carefully planned and reinforcing process, it hoped to present each future physician with an understanding of the role that he or she would play in the current clinical-socio-economic picture.

Awareness of cost outcomes for medical decision making encouraged the students to seek further knowledge and constantly to reevaluate prevailing medical practices. The students realized the logic of the integration of cost awareness into standard medical practice and education. They were made aware of the need for limits to, and the appropriate utilization of, advanced technology and the selective use of hospitalization.

The seminars were designed to acquaint the students with the responsibilities and interplay of the segments of society involved in health care: practicing physicians, patients, hospitals and other institutions, and governments. The cost-containment curriculum hoped to prepare the future physician for his or her new role as guardian of the public purse for medical care expenditures. The clinically oriented quality assurance and cost-containment program was more effective than previous programs based on seminars and group discussions of current events and issues. Integrating cost containment and quality assurance at the clinical level could not have been done without active support of the clinical faculty who served as role models for the students.

The following chapters describe in detail the objectives, methods, and evaluations of each educational approach. Each chapter can be treated as a module to be used singly or in concert with the others to fit most closely the time available and the educational needs of individual medical education settings. An integrated program that will reinforce itself at each level and become a logical part of medical education and decision making is encouraged.

REFERENCES

1. Gonnella, Joseph S., and Goran, M.J. "Quality of Patient Care—A Measurement of Change: The Staging Concept." *Medical Care* 13 (1976): 467.

2. Kessner, David M., Kalk, C.E., and Singer, J. "Assessing Health Care Quality—The Case for Tracers." *New Eng. J. Med.* 288:4 (January 25, 1973b): 189–194.

3. Kessner, Davis M., Kalk, C.E., and Singer, J. A *Strategy for Evaluating Health Services.* Institute of Medicine, National Academy of Sciences, Washington, D.C., 1973a.

4. National Commission on the Cost of Medical Care, Vols. I, II, and III, American Medical Association, Chicago, Illinois, 1977.

3   Chart Audit I

> I think [chart auditing] is a good method for making physicians aware of just how costly the diagnostic tests are. It also helps make us aware of exactly how we contribute to the tremendous and increasing cost of health care....
> —A student at the Medical College of Ohio, 1978

Analysis of health care through the review of patient records has been a cornerstone of health care evaluation since 1918, when the American College of Surgeons recommended medical record review as a standard of hospital practice. The recommendation was followed by the establishment of the Joint Commission on Accreditation of Hospitals (J.C.A.H.). Introduced and refined as a quality control method, chart review tacitly took on a cost containment role with the development of the Professional Standards Review Organizations (PSROs) in 1972. The PSROs were charged with determining the necessity, appropriateness, and quality of care in three ways: (1) validation of the justification for patients' hospitalization and length of stay, (2) study of medical practice profiles, and (3) audit of medical records.

Despite the prevalence of medical record review in the history of quality assurance activities, its effectiveness has been questioned: audits are only as good as the documentation in the medical record, and they frequently uncover no more than incomplete, illegible, or confusing notations on patients' charts.

Audits may be ineffective. Jessee (1977) complained that they do not result in "lasting changes in physician behavior or organization performance." Williamson charged that they "seem...to have had little documented impact in terms of improving patients' health...." Brook (1977) concluded that audits have "not contributed much to the goal of improving the health of the American people."

Part of the problem with chart auditing is the contradictory evidence regarding process and outcome measures of quality. Nobrega and others (1977) found "no correlation between the processes of medical care and the patient's outcome." Kane (1977), however, discovered that cases with good outcomes had better process scores than those with bad outcomes. Health care evaluators have had difficulty selecting specific process and outcome measures because medical practice and auditing of the same is not easy to control experimentally.

Audits are also very costly. According to Brook (1977), an estimated 50,000 audits were done by the J.C.A.H. in 1977 at a cost of $5,000 each. He commented that with an "annual expenditure of $250 million, assuring the quality of care is rapidly becoming a big business."

Audits often are "slow and cumbersome" and cost excessive physician time. They tend to focus on poor performance and "become a sterile activity performed solely for compliance purposes." They "suggest an academic, educational inquiry rather than a dynamic system that protects patients during their current episodes of care" (Vanagunas, 1979). Clearly, audits need to be refined and standardized both for their quality assurance and for their teaching value. It is precisely as an educational tool that audits can be adapted and presented to medical students, particularly in the teaching of cost-effective clinical management. It was as an attempt to reorganize audits into a standard teaching tool that the curriculum described below was developed.

DESCRIPTION OF CURRICULUM

The curriculum consisted of a series of four weekly seminars, each about 90 minutes long. The sessions included some discussion of the strengths and weaknesses of the various chart auditing methods, and such alternatives as mandatory continuing medical education for licensure and specialty recertification.

Each student received for auditing the complete medical record of a patient with hypertension or urinary tract infection. Hypertension and urinary tract infection cases were chosen for review because they were frequently encountered in the teaching hospitals. The students were provided with sets of previously defined explicit criteria for minimal care.

They audited the medical record according to four parameters.

1. the record system
2. the process of care
3. the patient's outcome
4. the cost of therapy

Each of the parameters was reported on by each student in completing the individual audits. They are outlined in Figure 3.1.

FIGURE 3.1. Instructions for chart review. Reprinted with permission from: Garg, M.L., Gliebe, W.A., Kleinberg, W.M.: "The Way We Teach Cost Containment," *Medical Teacher*, 2:5 (1980):222–228.

In his practice setting the student will audit the record of a patient with hypertension selected by his preceptor. The audit will analyze the record in four areas:

1. Record System
   (a) Organization of the record:
      (1) Clear and logical; problem or complaint-oriented.
      (2) Information easily retrievable.
      (3) Complete and up to date.
   (b) Legibility.

2. Process
   (a) Data base and workup optimal (using Phase 2 guidelines or Task Force on Hypertension Criteria, *Journal of the American Medical Association*, January 1977).
   (b) Each component of the data base:
      (1) Thorough.
      (2) Reliable.
      (3) Analytically logical.
      (4) Efficient.

3. Outcome
   (a) Determinants clear in assessment and plans.
   (b) Progress notes up-to-date and pertinent.
   (c) Patient's compliance and satisfaction accounted for.

4. Cost
   (a) Total cost of laboratory, radiographs and other tests from initial evaluation to present.
   (b) Cost if minimal care guidelines followed.
   (c) Discrepancies:
      (1) Define.
      (2) Positive, negative or no patient management.
   (d) Justification for.

Each student will prepare a report discussing all four areas, and the parameters described for each, for the record he reviewed. One typewritten page should follow, addressing the following:

1. Are discrepancies picked up by the chart audit and what accounts for them?
2. If there were cost differences, were they significant and could savings have been made without jeopardizing care?
3. Can chart audit be educational without being punitive?
4. What method of quality assurance would you prefer and why? (Refer to reference list.)
5. Can peer review through chart audit contain costs, save a physician time in his practice, and justify the time (and money) spent on auditing?
6. What are some other uses of chart audit besides feedback on individual patient care to physicians?

The Record System

The *objective of this component* was to make students aware of the importance of the retrievability of accurate patient data. Good record keeping is important not only because cases become increasingly more complicated, but also because of the new organizational patterns emerging in the practice of medicine. The latter include Health Maintenance Organizations, emergicenters, surgicenters, and hospital-sponsored neighborhood clinics. Physician continuity is often decreased in such practice arrangements, making effective record keeping a growing concern that needs to be stressed during the education program.

In their review of the record system, students were asked to check for legibility and organization to see if notations were clear, logical, complete, timely, and problem- or complaint-oriented. They also had to decide if information was easily retrieved.

Process and Outcome

The *objective of this component* was to familiarize students with the elements of process and outcome that can be measured to serve as indicators. A further objective was to find ways to determine the relationship between process and outcome. An assumption is made that this intervention (process), and its cost, produces some measurable improvement, and those interventions not contributing to improvement are extraneous. Unfortunately, it is not always clear in a clinical situation which decisions will be rewarding. Once a diagnosis is made with a high probability, it is easy to look back and see what did not contribute (using the "old retrospectoscope"). Much of the discussion of process and outcome deals with the justification of decisions, and the efficient, selective use of diagnostic tests and procedures. Frequently, many outcome criteria (e.g., relief of pain and suffering, reassurance, and satisfaction) are not documented. Another assumption is that efficient medical decision making reduces costs and results in the same outcome. Careful selection of diagnoses where there is a great consensus for the decision processes and where outcomes are well established makes the evaluation easier. Other conditions beg for more research and information before cost-benefit audits are meaningful.

During the analysis of process and outcome in medical records, students compared the actual process of care against minimal care plan criteria to determine if the patient's workup was thorough, reliable, logical, and efficient. They also studied progress notes, assessments, and patient-care-plans to judge if the outcome was apparent. It was also noted whether outcome took into consideration the patient's compliance and satisfaction.

Costs of Therapy

The objective of this component was to have students determine if any differences in cost were significant and had some effect, positive or negative, on patient management and outcome.

Students were asked to analyze cost by comparing the costs for laboratory, X ray, and other tests in the patient record against the total costs that would be incurred for necessary testing if Minimal Care Plan criteria were followed. It was recognized that the students were limited to standard textbook approaches in their analyses, but the discussions both emphasized justification of alternatives and were critical of decisions.

Students listed all the tests that had been performed on each hospital day. Then, with their assessments, students classified the tests as: useful and necessary; useful but not necessary; neither useful nor necessary. Students' classifications were given to a computer programmer who generated printouts showing the total number of tests and charges per day, the cumulative number of tests and charges per day, and the number of tests in each category per day.

The printout that was returned to the student provided him with a summary of the medical care process, the evaluation of the process as reflected in the tests ordered, and the costs of such appropriate or inappropriate care. The summary reflected the continual series of process—outcome steps inherent in medical treatment, reinforcing to the student how inappropriate "routine," "shotgun," or "cookbook" treatment strategies are for providing high-quality and cost-effective medical care.

The students could then suggest alternatives, such as having some tests done on an outpatient rather than inpatient basis. The extent to which alternatives could be defined provided another indicator of students' understanding of the complete health delivery system rather than one or two segments.

In the course of completing each component, students were addressing certain explicit objectives described above. To reinforce the need for an analytical approach to health care, students were asked to prepare concise responses, based on their previous work and the subjective and objective findings in the patient chart, to the following questions:

1. What was happening to the patient?
2. What was the problem?
3. What were the likely causes of the problems?
4. What other information, if any, was needed to delineate the problem and judge the patient's course?
5. Which tests were superfluous?
6. Which tests could have been replaced with less expensive or more reliable ones?
7. Cost of appropriate versus inappropriate care.

RESOURCE RECOMMENDATIONS

1. Faculty

   a. At least one member should be on the *clinical* faculty and be knowledgeable of the conditions being discussed; as many physicians as possible should be available to share in and rotate participation.
   b. At least one member should be familiar with health delivery systems, and with health economics and relevant public policy issues.
   c. Although computerized applications requiring a programmer on an as-needed basis have been used, these are not mandatory.

2. Materials

   a. Cooperation of the medical record department in developing materials that are anonymous, and protect patient confidentiality.
   b. Development of forms for students to expedite their work as much as possible.

3. Time

   a. Three to four seminar sessions to deal with the different components individually. The first session (if four are available) would be introductory, providing an issue overview and outlining specific assignments.
   b. A 90 minute seminar—two 40 minute segments separated by a ten minute break—for each session has been found effective.
   c. Seminars should be no more than two weeks apart to avoid unnecessary repetition for some students.
   d. Other departmental clinical faculty should be present when the *process and outcome* and *costs* components are scheduled. In the former, they can supplement the clinical discussion and review. In the latter, they can provide further credibility to consideration of the issue.

4. Number of Students and Space

   a. Assuming two faculty are involved regularly, about 12 students would be the desired maximum to facilitate discussion.
   b. A room that can facilitate group discussion; a room with a large table, or chairs in a circle, is suggested.

5. Evaluation

   a. The importance of the subject should be reflected in the overall grading process.
   b. Depending on chart audit's place in the overall curriculum, evaluation could include multiple-choice exam.
   c. If implemented during clinical clerkships, reinforcement of such concepts should be done during medical rounds. This

is why clinical-faculty support is so crucial to any significant program success. It is the cultivation of such role-model support that may be the most important step in program development.

6. Locus in Curriculum

Although the program may be implemented during the basic science or clinical segments, scheduling would be more problematic during the basic science segments. In addition, when students are studying basic science, they prioritize their work. Experience has shown that the importance of a subject is reflected in the enthusiasm and support given to it by the faculty and in its contribution to the student's grade.

Programs early and throughout the clinical curriculum would likely be optimal, since clinical behavior is then being moded. For practical scheduling reasons, two or more clinical departments should incorporate the program. For maximum support, faculty should be oriented to and prepared for the program well in advance. Faculty support and involvement would permit role-model and behavioral consistency to students.

Conclusion

Students reported that they were able to like "economics" lessons with patient care, thus assuring its "relevance." The mechanical portions of the activity were minimized, allowing students to avoid tedious tasks. Finally, by trying to touch future medical practices, this approach avoided the pitfalls of some other programs that address the social and political levels of "economics" and often become ideological debates with no positive lasting effect. After all, behavioral change is the goal of any educational program.

STUDENTS' COMMENTS

In reviewing the curricula offered at various times, we concluded that the reactions, comments and observations made by students would be useful to some educators contemplating similar cost-containment programs. Such feedback was used continually to adapt any current programs so that they might be more effective. Although student opinions were based on limited experience, and often superficial or rigid criteria, the discussions were useful to the development of a critical but flexible analytical process in the students. They demonstrated to the faculty the need for a continuing program to increase students' awareness and knowledge of the issues in medical economics.

In general, students found that they could audit any record so long as they understood the hospital record system in use. Students nevertheless preferred problem-oriented records. Problem-oriented records, they felt, were clear and logical and easier to review than source-oriented records. When "information is placed in the record according to the source from which it came (physicians, laboratory, X ray, nurses), the information is not easy to retrieve," said one student. Another said that in source-oreinted records, "the data are collected in a random fashion without any explanation as to why they were accumulated."

Even with problem-oriented records, students learned that analysis often could be hampered by incomplete or confusing notations. One student found that his problem-oriented record had a logical format and could be easily audited. However, the record lacked many important facts. The patient's diagnosis, condition, and vital signs were missing from the order sheet. Preoperative notes were not written. Progress notes did not have the physicians' interpretation of changes in the patient's condition, and the vital signs graphic sheet was incomplete.

Students decided that chart auditing could teach medical students and physicians to keep careful records which included the history, physical examination, plans of management, and follow-up studies. They agreed that systematic record keeping was essential for efficient auditing. It was also a time-saving device, since carefully recorded charts allowed physicians and other medical personnel to elicit data quickly. When care of a patient was transferred between physicians, good records reduced the risk of misinformation and duplication of services and increased efficiency of care.

Process and Outcome

Some students discovered that careful attention to the process of care did not always accompany concern for the treatment outcome. The workup of one patient was "optimal," said a student, because an intravenous pyelogram and voiding cystourethrogram were done promptly to rule out an anatomical defect as the basis for recurrent urinary-tract infection. The patient's brief period of hospitalization, in fact, "attests to the efficient execution of orders," the student said. "Other than a scheduled office visit in two weeks, however, there [was] simply a disregard for the outcome."

All laboratory tests for another patient were obtained efficiently so that "the patient's hospital stay was as brief as possible." However, the progress notes were

> very sketchy and did not include an assessment of the problem after the hospital workup was completed. The plans for follow-up were not clearly specified, [and] no mention was made concerning patient education, compliance, or satisfaction beyond the statement that the patient was to be seen in the doctor's office at some later date.

Cost of Therapy

Of the total of 201 tests done on the 12 patients in one audit, 155 tests were useful and necessary; they cost $1,898. However, 26 tests (costing $234) were judged useful but unnecessary, and 20 (costing $371) were judged unnecessary.

One student concluded that almost half of the patient's charges represented useless and unnecessary tests. The charges for the patient amounted to $234, but $122 was paid for tests that did not yield valuable information. The student felt that since the patient could have been treated as an outpatient, all hospital expenses could have been avoided. Criticism was made of an insurance program that covered only hospital expenses and not outpatient services.

Half of the cost of testing for another patient could have been saved, observed another student, by avoiding unnecessary tests. The total cost of testing for a 90-year-old woman who had been hospitalized "because she couldn't take care of herself... while arrangements were made for admission to a nursing home" was $247. The total cost of necessary tests, however, was only $124. During hospitalization, the woman had futile tests in response to vague complaints. She had blood cultures because she had "chills" but no spiking fevers. She had a skull series because of headaches, but she "never showed focal signs." She had liver enzyme analysis and a creatinine phosphokinase determination "for God knows what reason," said the student.

One four-year-old girl who had been hospitalized for recurrent urinary-tract infection had 15 laboratory tests and X rays, which cost $203.90. "Of these," said a student auditor, "there were seven useful and necessary tests which totaled $136.40." The remaining tests, which cost $67.50, "were not necessary to determine the final diagnosis." They were "useful since the patient was [to undergo] a procedure which required general anesthesia." Still, they could have been done on an outpatient basis, "thereby saving the... cost of another day of hospitalization."

One student who found a discrepancy between the actual cost of laboratory tests and the costs of necessary tests attributed the difference to the number of physicians involved in the care of the patient. The total cost of tests was $396; the cost of necessary tests was $319. Three of six urine cultures, one of three urinalyses, one blood urea nitrogen, a creatinine clearance, and a 24-hour urine collection for creatinine were not necessary. Said the student: "The fact that several orthopedic residents as well as urology consultants were caring for the patient may have been part of the reason more urine cultures were ordered than were really needed."

Are Audits Useful? The importance of their own experience could not help but impress upon students that hospital costs generated by physicians could be cut without reducing the quality of care. Many students praised the chart audit for uncovering costly, unnecessary tests. Remarked one student:

> I think [chart auditing] is a good method for making physicians aware of just how costly the diagnostic tests are. It also helps make us aware of exactly how we contribute to the tremendous and increasing cost of health care, indirectly by the use of lab tests that are not always useful or necessary. Peer review through chart audit should help contain costs by illustrating to physicians how 'routine admission orders' of tests, which may be useful but not necessary, add to costs.

Some students thought chart auditing could help to contain health care costs by acting as a "deterrent to physicians [who] inflate [their] bills by ordering useless tests" or by picking up trends of unnecessary hospital admissions and diagnostic procedures. Others, however, felt that "the costs of review could easily outrun the benefits, [especially] if the review program became too big and expensive." "It is doubtful," one student stated, " that chart auditing can pay for itself in our present health care system. Although costs probably could be contained, the savings would be negligible compared to the expenditure needed to run the bureaucracy born from chart audit." Another pointed out that "unless people are punished in some manner, and continuing education is encouraged, merely the auditing of charts will do little to contain costs or justify the time and money spent on chart audit."

Keeping the control of health care evaluation in the hands of medical professionals is, perhaps, one reason why students preferred hospital-based audit programs to regional review by PSROs. One student observed:

> The PSRO approach is looking at the situation from the angle of the patient's needs via the health care delivery system, and this is truly important.... [However], the PSRO deals with services to the patient with [little] regard to the physician's predicament as to which care approach is the best for the patient. [In contrast], patient care audit...at the hospital level seems to be set up to assist physicians by encouraging reassessment [through] medical education.

Said another: "Review supervised by peers at a local level seems preferable to me. This would keep the bureaucracy as small as possible and permit easier input into the system. Such a system would be more responsive to local needs and conditions."

Students also preferred auditing systems that included both process and outcome measures, and concentrated on using audit findings for continuing medical education activities. A student observed that chart auditing could help plan CME "so past experience with particular problems can be used to...solve those same problems when they reappear.... [Learning] the number and frequency of problems in a physician's patient population can help the physician to concentrate his continuing education on these problems." The student had unwittingly elaborated on Clement Brown's (1973) bicycle concept of continuing medical education!

Students decided that chart auditing could be used as a teaching device in medical school and as a means for encouraging health care professionals to organize their records more effectively. "The chart audit also [could] be used to improve the thoroughness of history-taking and physical examination techniques, to enhance [physicians'] analytic sense, and thereby to [increase] overall efficiency [in] time, cost, and energy."

REFERENCES

1. Brook, R.H. "Quality. Can We Measure It?" *New Eng. J. Med.* 296 (January 20, 1977): 170.

2. Brown, Clement R. "Assessing Quality of Care—The Bicycle Concept." In *The Hospital's Role in Assessing the Quality of Medical Care—Proceedings of the 15th Annual Symposium on Hospital Affairs—May, 1973.* Edited by Scheye, E. University of Chicago Press, 1973.

3. Jessee, W.F. "Quality Assurance Systems: Why Aren't There Any?" *Quality Rev. Bull.* 3 (November 1977): 16.

4. Kane, R.L., et al. "Relationship between Process and Outcome in Ambulatory Care. *Medical Care.* 15 (November 1977): 961.

5. Nobrega, F.T., et al. "Quality Assessment in Hypertension: Analysis of Process and Outcome Methods." *New Eng. J. Med.* 296 (January 20, 1977): 145.

6. Vanagunas, Anbdrone. "Quality Assessment: Alternate Approaches." *Quality Rev. Bull.* 5 (February 1979): 7–10.

7. Williamson, John W., "Evaluating Quality of Patient Care—A Strategy Relating Outcome and Process Assessment." *JAMA* 218:4 (1971): 564–569.

4
Chart Audit II: Tracers and Staging

Health care evaluation is still a new and rudimentary discipline.
—John R. Hogness, President
Institute of Medicine

The Institute of Medicine (1973) adapted the concept of tracers from physiology and nuclear medicine for its extensive study to assess the quality of medical care. Similarly, the ideas about staging a disease to form comparable clusters were adapted by Gonnella and Goran (1975) from oncology. These two concepts became the starting points for the earliest quality assurance education programs developed and implemented.

The Tracer Method of Evaluating Health Care

A tracer is a well recognized, measurable condition whose course (and outcome) can be followed readily and analyzed, and whose course helps to measure the function of the system in which it is present. Kessner, et al. (1973), proposed looking at illnesses that could be used like tracers to "shed...light on how particular parts of the (health) system work, not in isolation, but in relation to one another...."

The tracer method was designed to measure both processes and outcomes of care because "it is impossible to pinpoint the strengths and weaknesses of process without knowing the outcome, but outcome alone can be misleading if the patient receives unnecessary diagnostic tests or inappropriate treatment" (Kessner et al., 1973).

The methodology identified six characteristics of a disease entity in order to qualify as a tracer:

33

1. "A tracer should have a definite functional impact."

2. It should be "relatively well defined and easy to diagnose."

3. A tracer's prevalence rate "should be high enough to permit the collection of adequate data from a limited population sample."

4. A tracer's natural history "should vary with the utilization and effectiveness of medical care," so that the progress of the tracer disease is truly altered by health services.

5. "The techniques of medical management... should be well defined for... prevention, diagnosis, treatment, or rehabilitation," at least according to minimal, agreed upon standards.

6. "The effects of nonmedical factors on the tracer should be understood" so that social, cultural, economic, behavioral, and environmental factors are not responsible for changes in prevalence or distribution of the disease.

Six disease conditions were identified that fulfilled the six criteria. These were: middle ear infection and hearing loss, visual disorders, iron-deficiency anemia, cervical cancer, hypertension, and urinary-tract infection. The latter two tracers were used in developing the curriculum at the Medical College of Ohio.

DESCRIPTION OF CURRICULUM

Both tracers selected offer certain health-care evaluation opportunities:

> An adequate evaluation of the patient with an elevated blood pressure will reflect not only the quality of the general history and physical examination but, specifically, those aspects related to the cardiovascular system. It will provide an opportunity to assess the appropriate use of laboratory tests and will reveal much about the manner in which drugs are used....
>
> [Proper management of] both asymptomatic and symptomatic urinary-tract infection requires a careful history, selected physical examination, and a good understanding of the limitations of commonly used laboratory procedures.... [Also,] because a variety of

antimicrobial drugs, many with potentially serious side effects, is available for treatment, this tracer provides a discriminating tool for assessing the use of this common class of drugs.... (Kessner et al., 1973)

One *objective* of studying these two tracer conditions was to let students focus on proper history-taking and physical examinations and the use of appropriate laboratory tests and drugs for many of the patients they saw during their clinical rotations.

Another *objective* in setting up a series of clinical curriculum seminars was to teach students about the tracer methodology and adapt it to teach them about assessing the quality and cost of medical care.

As part of a series of four seminars, students were first asked to read the general background chapter and the specific chapters on hypertension and urinary-tract infection in *A Strategy for Evaluating Health Services* (Kessner et al., 1973). For the second seminar, students were divided into groups of four and asked to set criteria for the management of the tracer conditions. The difficulties and limitations of tracers were also discussed.

Kessner recognized that objective evaluation of health care is impossible without criteria for comparison, so he formulated sets of criteria, called Minimal Care Plans, for each of his six selected tracers. These criteria were designed to "outline baseline care [and to be] pragmatic, taking into account the unavailability of sophisticated diagnostic equipment."

Tracers in Hypertension

For hypertension, the Minimal Care Plan included 12 specific items under history, and seven under physical examination (Figure 4.1). Criteria for history-taking covered the symptoms that physicians should inquire about, that is, chest pain, foot edema, shortness of breath, paroxysmal nocturnal dyspnea, and orthopnea.

During a later seminar, students examined the charts of two selected patients with hypertension to analyze the cost of care. Their objectives were to determine the cost of the Minimal Care Plan for the treatment of hypertension and compare it with the cost of care that had been provided. They also intended to find out the common deviations from the Minimal Care Plan and decide if the deviations had any effect on the management or outcome of patients.

FIGURE 4.1. A minimal care plan for hypertension. Reproduced from "A Strategy for Evaluating Health Services," 1973, with the permission of the National Academy Press, Washington, DC 20418.

I. Screening

    A. Method. The systolic pressure is recorded at the onset of the first Korotkoff sound, and the diastolic at the final disappearance of the second or the change if the sound persists.

    B. Criteria. An individual patient is judged in need of evaluation for elevated blood pressure if the mean of three or more systolic or diastolic pressures exceeds the age-specific criteria specified below:

MALES & FEMALES	SYSTOLIC	DIASTOLIC
18–44 years	140	90
45–64 years	150	95
65 or older	160	95

II. Evaluation

In the evaluation of elevated blood pressure, the history and physical examination data listed below should be obtained early in the evaluation.

    A. History. (1) Personal and social history; (2) family history of high blood pressure, coronary-artery disease, or stroke; (3) previous diagnosis of high blood pressure (females, toxemia of pregnancy or pre-eclampsia) and time of first occurrence; (4) previous treatment for high blood pressure (when started and when stopped, and drugs used); (5) chest pain, pressure, or tightness; location, length of symptoms, frequency of symptoms, effect of deep breathing, description of feeling (crushing, smothering, strangling), symptom temporarily curtails activity and pain radiates into left shoulder, arm, or jaw and is accompanied by nausea, shortness of breath or fast or fluttering heart beat; (6) feet swell; (7) shortness of breath; (8) patient awakens wheezing or feeling smothered or choked; (9) patient sleeps on two or more pillows; (10) prior history of kidney trouble, nephrosis or nephritis; (11) history of kidney infection; and (12) prior X ray examination of kidneys.

    B. Physical Examination. (1) Weight and height; (2) blood pressure—supine and up-right; (3) funduscopic; (4) heart—abnormal sounds or rhythm; (5) neck—thyroid and neck veins; (6) abdomen—standard description, including abdominal bruit; and (7) extremities—peripheral pulses and edema.

C. Laboratory. (1) Urinalysis; (2) hematocrit or hemoglobin; and (3) blood urea nitrogen or serum creatinine.

D. Other Tests. (1) Electrocardiogram, if the patient is less than 30 years of age or if diastolic pressure is 130 mm of mercury or greater; and (2) rapid-sequence intravenous pyelogram.

III. Diagnosis

A. Essential Hypertension. As described above under I.B. (Criteria), provided there is no evidence of secondary hypertension.

B. Secondary Hypertension. Hypertension secondary to renal, adrenal, thyroid, or primary vascular disease.

IV. Management
All drugs are prescribed in acceptable dosages adjusted to the individual patient, contraindications are observed, and patients are monitored for common side effects according to the information detailed in AMA Drug Evaluations 1971 (first edition). Fixed-dosage combinations should not be used for initial therapy.

A. Mild Essential Hypertension (Diastolic Pressure of 115 mm of mercury). (1) Initial treatment with thiazides alone in a diuretic dose; (2) if pressure is not reduced by 10 mm of mercury or to lowest level that patient can tolerate without symptoms of hypotension in two to four weeks, alpha-methyldopa, reserpine or hydralazine is added to thiazide.

B. Moderate Essential Hypertension (Diastolic Pressure of 115 to 130 mm of mercury). (1) Initial treatment with thiazide and alpha-methyldopa, reserpine, or hydralazine; (2) if no response after two to four weeks change to thiazide-reserpine-hydralazine or thiazide-guanethidine combination.

C. Severe Essential Hypertension (Diastolic Pressure of 130 mm of mercury of Keith-Wagener Grade III or IV Funduscopic Changes). Refer to specialist or hospitalize (or both).

D. Secondary Hypertension. Treat, or refer for treatment of, primary condition.

E. Undetermined Etiology or No Response to Treatment. Hypertension of undetermined cause or not responding to treatment regimen above requires further evaluation, to include: (1) determination of serum sodium and potassium; and, if not previously performed, (2) rapid-sequence intravenous pyelography.

Students checked the current cost of drugs, laboratory tests, and X rays in the MCO Hospital pharmacy, laboratories, and radiology department. They analyzed the diagnostic and therapeutic management of patients by thoroughly reviewing the records of patients who had been identified as hypertensive on the Outpatient Clinics' composite patient lists.

Tracers in Urinary-Tract Infection

In similar studies of urinary-tract infection, students compared Kessner's Minimal Care Plan (Figure 4.2) against the treatment of 21 outpatients and 25 inpatients at the teaching hospitals and clinics. They discovered that all outpatient records met the Minimal Care Plan criteria for history-taking, physical examination, and necessary laboratory work (urinalysis and microscopic examination of sediment). They discovered that a complete blood count was the most common deviation from the Minimal Care Plan, but they failed to "see how it added to the diagnosis or treatment of urinary-tract infection." Students did see that it added to the costs. Another deviation was intravenous pyelograms (IVPs). Students discovered that two women had IVPs which "were not clearly indicated" by the Minimal Care Plan. The unnecessary IVPs added significantly to the cost.

Another group of students tabulated the cost of hospital care of

FIGURE 4.2. A minimal care plan for urinary tract infection. Reproduced from "A Strategy for Evaluating Health Services," 1973, with the permission of the National Academy Press, Washington, DC 20418.

I. Screening

    A. Quantitative urine culture. (1) Pregnant women: once each trimester; (2) females: yearly, if history of previous urinary-tract infections; (3) males and females with hypertension.

II. Evaluation (Initial Episode of Symptomatic or Asymptomatic Significant Bacteriuria)

    A. History. (1) Presenting complaint; (2) previous bladder or kidney infection or kidney stone; (3) previous history of instrumentation or surgery (if yes, specify the date); (4) present history of dysuria, hematuria, frequency, nocturia; (5) pain (if yes, specify location: groin, lower abdomen, costovertebral angle (CVA), genitalia); (6) fever, chills; (7) history of previous treatment for this episode.

B. Physical examination. (1) Temperature; (2) blood pressure; (3) palpation of abdomen with reference to suprapubic and CVA regions; (4) genitalia (external genital exam for females); (5) rectal (males only).

C. Laboratory (in addition to quantitative urine culture). Clean voided urine specimen for routine analysis and microscopic examination of sediment.

III. Management

A. Criteria for treatment. (1) Treat all patients with 100,000 colonies per ml of any pathogenic organism; (2) with symptoms of sepsis or bacteria on unspun urine sediment, treat prior to results of quantitative culture; (3) less than 10,000 colonies per ml of any organism and no history of previous treatment: no treatment indicated; (4) 10,000–100,000 colonies per ml of any pathogenic organism: require three positive quantitative cultures before treating.

B. Hospitalization with initial infection indicated: (1) If patient is acutely ill on presentation as indicated by presence of sepsis (fever, sweat, prostration, chills) or by being too ill to come to physician's office without help; (2) where obstruction is present as well as infection; (3) where infection is accompanied by renal failure.

C. Office treatment indicated. The patient who is uncomfortable, but not septic, and can pass urine should be treated as an outpatient.

D. Treatment. (1) Symptomatic treatment for dysuria without evidence of bacterial infection; (2) antibacterial treatment.
All drugs are prescribed in acceptable dosages adjusted to the individual patient, contraindications are observed, and patients are monitored for common side effects according to information detailed in AMA Drug Evaluations, 1971. Fixed-dosage combinations should not be used for initial therapy.
Initial treatment with a soluble sulfonamide, tetracycline, ampicillin, or nitrofurantoin. If within 48 hours the symptoms do not respond to the first drug, alternative drug therapy should be initiated. Duration of antimicrobial treatment: 7–14 days.

E. Follow-up. (1) Repeat urine culture one week after treatment is stopped; (2) intravenous pyelogram (IVP) for history of infection during childhood, more than two episodes in females, and after first episode in males.

F. Referral. (1) To urologist if there is IVP evidence of genitourinary anomaly or obstruction; (2) to specialist for treatment of persistent and resistant bacterial infection in the absence of genitourinary anomaly or obstruction.

urinary-tract infection by age, specialty of the attending physician, and length of stay. Students confined their cost analysis to laboratory investigations and X rays, carefully studying the charts of patients with the highest and lowest charges.

Variations of individual cases were dealt with in detail by the students, looking to the clinical data for explanations. They served as the essential bridge, when teaching cost effectiveness, to actual medical practice. The bridge is perhaps the most important one to maintain when trying to keep students' motivation and receptiveness at acceptable levels.

The Staging Concept

With pathological, anatomical, and physiological findings, oncologists classify the extent of a patient's disease so that they can predict the outcome of therapy. Through staging, they group similar patients in order to choose the mode of therapy most likely to succeed and to compare the results of treatment with other patients in different cancer centers.

Staging also can be an assessment tool in quality assurance. It classifies patients by the severity of their disease to:

> identify...groups or clusters of patients [who] require common treatment and services and have similar outcomes [so that health-care evaluators can] compare the results of care for patients with conditions of similar severity (Gonnella and Goran, 1975).

By determining the stage of disease at a particular point in the treatment of an outpatient, "the seriousness of the patient's condition ...[could be] a good indicator" of the treatment that had gone before. Admittedly, "potential causes of the severity of a problem include the willingness of the patient to seek medical attention early...or the natural evolution of the problem in that particular patient." It also, however, can reflect the "availability of medical care, the clinical judgement of the physician, [and] the setting in which care is provided" (Gonnella, et al., 1976).

Since a major criticism of Kessner's tracer method by students was its failure to consider the severity of disease, the staging concept was introduced into the curriculum at the Medical College of Ohio. Staging might permit a more realistic view of the complexities of disease and the many problems that often afflict patients. The staging plan might also reduce the time spent by students in chart review, because once the stages of a disease have been set by health-care professionals, the task of classifying individual patients' disease severity can be done by clerical personnel or even by computer. The faculty thought that staging in combination with a Minimal Care Plan would help students gain a better understanding of the diagnosis and treatment of hypertension, and give them experience in judging the adequacy of patient management.

Students in groups of four were asked to follow the staging approach to health-care analysis and classify hypertension into three stages on the basis of severity: Stage I, which included mild disease with no complications; Stage II, which included moderately severe disease with local complications; and Stage III, which included serious disease with systemic complications.

With Gonnella and Goran's (1975) staging of hypertension (Figure 4.3) as a guide and the advice of a consultant cardiologist, students defined mild, moderate, and severe states of hypertension and developed a Minimal Care Plan for each stage (Figure 4.4). Students then compared

FIGURE 4.3. Disease stages. Reprinted with permission from Gonnella, J.S., and Goran, M.J., "Quality of patient Care—A Measurement of Change: The Staging Concept," *Medical Care* 13 (1975).

Diseases	Stage 1 (No Complications)	Stage 2 (Local Complications)	Stage 3 (Systemic Complications)
ESSENTIAL HYPERTENSION	Essential Hypertension— minimal (diastolic pressure equal to or less than 110 mm Hg)	Essential Hypertension— moderate (diastolic pressure equal to or less than 140 mm Hg)	Essential Hypertension— severe (diastolic pressure greater than 140 mm Hg) with one or more complications; papilledema; cerebral-vascular accident; uremia; hypertensive heart disease manifested by congestive heart failure

FIGURE 4.4. Staging and Minimal Care Plan.

Staging and Minimal Care Plan

CRITERIA: Patient must have elevated blood pressure on three or more occasions. Elevated BP is defined as being greater than 140/90 if patient is less than 45 years of age, and greater than 150/95 for 45 years and over.

Stages

I	II	III
Mild Essential Hypertension (90–110 mmHg. diastolic)	*Moderate Essential Hypertension* (110–130 mmHg. diastolic)	*Severe Essential Hypertension* (<130 mmHg. diastolic)
A. Mild increase in blood pressure without symptoms and clinical findings.	A. Moderate increase of BP without other clinical findings.	A. Severe increase of BP with retinopathy through Stage IV without other obvious organ involvement.
B. Mild increase in blood pressure with A/V nicking and narrow but no other obvious organ involvement.	B. Moderate increase of BP with only Stage I – III retinopathy.	B. Severe increase of BP with any combination of clinically evident renal, neurological, cardiac or vascular compromise.
	C. Moderate increase of BP with EKG or radiological evidence of LVH.	

History
(same for all three Stages)

In addition to information elicited in a routine history, the following items are considered as essential to assess hypertension in the patient.

1. Family history of hypertension, early death, myocardial infarctions, diabetes, hyperlipoproteinemias.
2. History of previous diagnosis, treatment, and response in patient of hypertension.
3. Incidence of dyspnea, syncope, shortness of breath, paroxysmal nocturnal dyspnea, orthopnea, headaches, blurred vision, intermittent claudication, strokes, transient ischemic attacks; angina pectoris, hyperlipoproteinemia, myocardial infarction, medications patient is taking, especially estrogens as pills, diuretics, thyroid replacement, bronchodilators, and mood elevators.
4. History of diabetes, thyroid disease toxemia of pregnancy in patient.
5. History of headache, perspiration, palpation, tremor, anxiety, facial pallor, weight loss.
6. History of weakness, paresthesia, paralysis, nausea, polyuria, nocturia, polydipsia, chest pain.
7. History of renal disease, proteinuria, hematuria.
8. History of developing frontal baldness, truncal obesity, loss of libido, and abdominal striae, increased bruising.
9. History of epistaxis.
10. History of smoking.

Physical Examination
(same for all three Stages)

In addition to a routine examination, the following are essential to a work-up for hypertension.

1. General appearance — blood pressure both arms lying and standing. Note height, weight, obesity, and its distribution, striae, ecchymoses, xanthelasma, tremor, excessive perspiration, frontal baldness.
2. Head and neck — thorough funduscopic examination after pupils have been dilated. Thyroid adequately palpated.
3. Auscultation of lungs.
4. Cardiovascular — heart evaluation should include point of PMI, rhythm, S-4, S-3, murmurs, thrills. Bruits should be listened for in carotids, supraclavicular spaces, abdomen, and flanks. Jugular venous distension is evaluated and peripheral pulses assessed.
5. Neurological exam should include checking for hyperreflexia, incoordination, any areas of parethesis.
6. Edema, cyanosis, and other signs of compromised peripheral perfusion.

43

FIGURE 4.4. *(continued)*

Stages

I Mild Essential Hypertension (90–110 m m Hg. diastolic)	II Moderate Essential Hypertension (110–130 m m Hg. diastolic)	III Severe Essential Hypertension (<130 m m Hg. diastolic)

Laboratory
(same for all three Stages)

The following include the data needed for an initial minimal assessment.
1. Electrocardiogram.
2. Chest X ray—PA and lateral.
3. Urine analysis.
4. Complete blood count with hematocrit and hemoglobin.
5. Serum Na, K, Cl, CO_2, BUN, creatinine, uric acid.
6. Fasting blood sugar.
7. Cholesterol and triglycerides.

Management

I	II	III
A. (1) Initial treatment with diuretics, i.e. Thiazides alone, dose up to 100 mg. hydrochlorthiazide or equivalent. (2) In 2–4 weeks, add on a mild antihypertensive agent if BP has not decreased by 10 mm Hg. May need longer period to adjust diet, weight.	A. Treat as in Stage I. B. Begin patient on diuretic along with a mild antihypertensive agent. Titrate this agent up to maximal dose over 1–3 month period before adding another antihypertensive agent. Include items 3–5 in Stage I treatment plan.	A. (1) With acute symptomatic patient treat with parenternal antihypertensive. (2) Hospitalize all patients with newly discovered severe essential hypertension for appropriate assessment and until control of blood pressure is maintained.

44

(3) Give K-replacement as needed.
(4) Follow patient every two weeks until stable and then every 3–6 months, with electrolytes, urinalysis, blood pressure, funduscopic and cardiovascular exam.
(5) Instruct patient about course of the disease and complications associated with smoking, obesity, and moderate Na restriction.

C. Treatment is same as for B.

(3) Treat patient with diuretics and either combination antihypertensive agents or a single strong agent as guanethidine.
(4) Again complete items 3–5 in Stage I treatment plan.

B. (1) Hospitalize patient for BP control and to assess organ damage.
(2) In addition to the initial workup the following should be obtained:
24 hour urinary creatinine and protein creatinine clearance, rapid sequence IVP, serum total protein, urinary electrolytes.
(3) Treat appropriately any complications of organ involvement.

45

the records of hypertensive patients against the Minimal Care Plan criteria to judge:

1. The adequacy of diagnosis and management of the patient's problems.

2. The efficacy of diagnostic and therapeutic programs based on the time it took to evaluate the patient and the choice of the most likely tests to reach a conclusion in a reasonable length of time.

3. The economy of treatment based on its costs and the convenience to the patient.

In the review of patient records, students rated the quality of health care by staging the patient's condition and then grading the history, physical examination, diagnostic plan, treatment, and patient education. Finally, students determined the patient's outcome and the factors that might affect it (see Figure 4.5 for students' instructions).

FIGURE 4.5. Instructions for chart audit.

---

1. Identify disease stage of the patient according to the definition developed by your class.

2. Identify key pertinent positive and negative items in the medical history and see if they are present.

3. Identify tracer condition (as defined by Kessner and Kalk in the *New England Journal of Medicine*) and examine chart for presence of the tracer. Do you feel that the tracer concept is helpful in defining patients' evaluation by physicians?

4. Identify key pertinent physical findings related to the diagnosis and see if they are present in the record.

5. Determine if adequate assessment is recorded and if the assessment is backed up by the subjective and objective recordings.

6. Determine if minimal diagnostic workup (according to your protocol) has been initiated.

7. Determine if adequate therapy (according to your protocol) has been initiated.

8. Determine if adequate patient education has been carried out and if follow-up visits have been planned.

9. Using the table below, record your audit findings according to the scale provided.

Patient #	Stage	(A) History	(B) Physical	(C) Diagnostic	(D) Treatment	(E) Education	(F) Outcome
1							
2							
3							
4							

SCALE:

For (A) to (E)	For Outcome
1. Excellent	1. Optimal Result
2. Average or good	2. Could have been improved
3. Below average	3. Minimal desired
4. Poor	4. Poor
5. Indeterminate	5. Indeterminate

10. Can you determine outcome of the patient's care from your audit?

RESOURCE RECOMMENDATIONS FOR TRACERS AND STAGING

1. Faculty

   a. At least one member should be a clinical professor; as many physicians as possible should be involved at least as faculty advisors on assignments.
   b. Some support from public health or social sciences faculty, particularly during the first session when the conceptual underpinnings of further assignments are being developed.

2. Materials

    a. Cooperation of medical records department to provide students limited access to selected cases.
    b. A curriculum binder containing relevant readings that can be reused (for economic reasons and because new articles are added regularly). The course outline is included at the front for one time use. This is distributed to participating students at least five days before the first meeting.

3. Time

    a. Three to four seminars, the first being introductory and establishing the basis for the remaining sessions. The second seminar focuses on criteria development while the third and fourth (sometimes combined) deal primarily with the results of field studies.
    b. The first seminar needs about 90 minutes, the second about two hours and the last (if merged) also about two hours.
    c. Seminars are scheduled over one-month clerkship, one week apart.

4. Number of Students and Space

    a. Seminar size of about 12 would be best to allow working subgroups, comparison of results, and personalized discussion.

5. Evaluation

    a. In addition to evaluating assignments and participation, clinical faculty should be observing students' behavior in clinics.
    b. Evaluation of their clinical behavior before and after the seminar could also be useful. Since this would be time consuming, it could be done periodically and randomly to yield data on the impact of the program.

6. Locus in Curriculum

The program is best included in the clinical curriculum where application of new knowledge and correlation with clinical cases helps reinforce the concepts.

CONCLUSIONS

The development and study of staging increased students' awareness of early case finding and primary prevention. Gonnella and Goran's (1975) work with staging has stressed the need for preventive medicine and changes in lifestyle as a means of reducing the cost of medical care. As several studies have indicated, medical problems that are diagnosed in Stage I are less expensive to manage since there are fewer complications. The students' analyses bore this out. They discovered that diagnostic and treatment costs rose with the stage of the disease, and they concluded that patients with easy access to health services and good medical follow-up will pay less in both money and morbidity.

While tracer and staging have severe limits in quality of care assessment, they are a complex, sophisticated learning tool for medical students and resident physicians. Developing Minimal Care Plans and staging disease enhanced the students' understanding of hypertension and the importance of the history, physical examination, and the diagnostic, therapeutic, and educational plans on the patient's outcome and dollar costs to the health system.

STUDENTS' COMMENTS

In preparing their own Minimal Care Plan, at least one group of students felt that the Kessner criteria were inadequate. The students pointed out that since cerebrovascular disease is a major cause of death from hypertension, neurologic symptoms should also be investigated. The group felt that Kessner's criteria for examination of the heart during the physical were not specific enough. The students believed that the criterion "abnormal heart sounds and rhythm" should be replaced by descriptions of the first and second heart sounds and include the heart rate.

Students' Minimal Care Plan for hypertension included three "necessary" tests: urinalysis, hemoglobin or hematocrit, and blood urea nitrogen (BUN or serum creatinine determination). Taking into account the possible need for other tests on hypertensives, students listed on the Minimal Care Plan electrocardiogram and infusion intravenous pyelogram for patients under age 30 or older patients with diastolic pressure over 130 mm Hg.

The actual cost of testing in the Outpatient Clinics ranged from the minimum office call fee for one patient who had not had tests performed, to full cost for a patient who had urinalysis, serum electrolytes, complete blood count, infusion IVP, chest X ray, and EKG. The average cost of diagnostic testing for hypertensive patients, however, was 33 percent higher than the cost of the Minimal Care Plan.

After the students' changes had been made in the Minimal Care Plan, two evaluations needed to be done for subsequent seminars. The first dealt with quality. Students analyzed the workups that had been done on 19 hypertensive clinic patients. In their review of patient records, the students found that the histories and physicals were inferior. Only two of the 13 criteria for history taking on the Minimal Care Plan were consistently reported: patient complaints of shortness of breath and previous diagnosis of hypertension. All others were ignored. Personal and social histories were either omitted, or merely included "a line or two about smoking habits and marital status." One of the patients who had been treated for hypertension at the Clinic for two years had been hospitalized four years earlier for treatment of hydronephrosis and pyelonephritis. The students found that "there was [no] comment made about this in the chart in the subsequent two years." Outcomes differed because patients failed to comply with medication or dietary regimens.

Students considered physical examination of the optic fundi as the key to the clinical evaluation of hypertensive vascular disease; yet the condition of the fundi was seldom described. "It is difficult to believe that such an important aspect of an exam is omitted so frequently," they reported. "One must assume that the problem is just failure to report a negative exam. If not, [the] clinics are giving much less than minimal care."

At the final seminar in the series on the tracer methodology, students discussed the value of the Minimal Care Plan in assessing the quality of care. Students said that the exercise gave them the chance to learn about Minimal Care Plans and to gain an insight into the treatment and cost of care of hypertension and urinary-tract infection. Students noted, however, that the Joint Commission on Quality Assurance in Ambulatory Care, which included representatives from major medical specialty societies, could agree on minimum care criteria for only six of 60 diagnostic categories. Even if minimal criteria for many tracer conditions could be set, the wide variations in diagnostic plans and management of non-tracer diseases make judgments about the care offered in a community tenuous at best.

One group of students felt that the outcome for one 63-year-old man was "bleak," because he consistently failed to comply with his medication schedules and to keep his clinic appointments. The man had Stage III hypertension which had caused several hospitalizations; yet students found that "there [was] not a complete history or physical in his clinic chart" and it appeared that "no one had done a complete evaluation of [the patient's] hypertension" in the past eight years. "The multitude of tests ordered [during that time] gives an adequate data base. However, the pertinent lab tests should have been ordered when [the patient] was initially diagnosed." As a consequence of inadequate evaluation, treatment of the patient's hypertension was ineffective, and the patient's blood pressure remained high.

Another group of students decided that, although a patient had a good or average history, physical, and diagnostic evaluation, the physician "in charge of the case did not rule out the anxiety reaction as a cause of high blood pressure." This patient had Stage III hypertension but "no past history of high blood pressure and no [complaints] of fainting spells, chest pain, or dyspnea.... [The patient] did have a history of headaches with nervousness and some sweating." The students questioned why the physician did not conduct a systems review and why certain tests were ordered. They believed that the physician "jumped to ruling out carcinoid syndrome and hyperthyroidism by ordering appropriate tests for [them but] with no real evidence that these were clinical impressions."

Students decided that the outcome of another patient was poor because the treatment did not consider the patient's convenience. Medication for one patient who had Stage II hypertension was "begun on the first visit after [diagnostic] studies were complete. [However,] its continuation was sporadic. [The patient continued] to show elevated blood pressure on each visit, but medication was not...increased or changed...." Even though the patient had "frequently missed her appointments and explained that she was unable to come to the clinic that often, no arrangements were made to improve the situation or to make certain that [the patient] had enough medication to last until she would be able to visit the clinic."

After the record review, most of the students agreed that the use of the Minimal Care Plan had taught them the value of establishing standards of medical practice and had given them the incentive to keep up with current knowledge in medicine. One student remarked that he had become aware of the difficulties involved in peer review by trying to set up an explicit set of criteria for the Minimal Care Plan.

Other students spoke of particular problems with tracers or staging. One noted that

> as a time-saving device, the tracer concept [is] quite valuable.... Since careful recording of medical histories, physical exams, plans of management, and follow-up studies are essential to the future care of patients in busy hospitals and outpatient departments, the tracer is also valid as an assessment of the quality of medical care....
>
> The use of hypertension as a tracer, however, presented some problems. The establishment of disease stages to assess adequacy of treatment was useless. Unless the patient is first worked up at a given institution or fails to comply with a therapeutic regimen, he is already being managed for the disease, and true diastolic levels are difficult to obtain. Adequate treatment could thus be judged only by the patient's outcome.... If disease staging is to be useful in this assessment, staging of the disease must be based on criteria other than blood pressure levels themselves.

After finding several general areas of deficiency in the chart audit, a student wondered

> whether these [deficiencies] represent omission in the actual workup or merely failure to record appropriate information.... It would seem that many of these deficiencies would be overcome if standards were set up for the...clinics whereby each student or physician would know precisely what information must be sought and recorded. The appropriateness of treatment follow-up and outcome could be much more thoroughly assessed using this condition as a tracer.

However, many students pointed out that the standardization of diagnosis and treatment should not be allowed to stifle innovative practices.

Students believed that the concept of the tracer condition is valid and effective only in regard to a specific disease, and they observed that it would be dangerous to extrapolate the findings for one tracer condition to assess the overall quality of health care delivered in a clinic or hospital. They found that staging can improve the reliability of chart auditing, but it does not reduce the time needed to process the data. Clerical personnel could stage a patient's disease, but health care professionals still had to scrutinize all facts in the patient's chart to make judgments about the quality of care.

REFERENCES

1. Gonnella, J.S., and Goran, M.J. "Quality of Patient Care—A Measurement of Change: The Staging Concept." *Med. Care* 13 (1975): 467.

2. Gonnella, J.S., Louis, D.Z., and McCord, J.J. "The Staging Concept—An Approach to Assessment of Outcome of Ambulatory Care." *Med. Care* 14 (1976): 13.

3. Kessner, David M., Kalk, C.E., and Singer, J. "Assessing Health Care Quality—The Case for Tracers." *New Eng. J. Med.* 288:4 (January 25, 1973): 189–194.

4. Kessner, David M., and Kalk, C.E. *A Strategy for Evaluating Health Services.* Institute of Medicine, National Academy of Sciences, Washington, D.C., 1973.

5

Chart Audit III: Preadmission Testing

One hint I would give to all who attend or visit the sick, to all who have to pronounce an opinion upon sickness or its progress. Come back and look at your patient after he has had an hour's animated conversation with you.

—Florence Nightingale, 1859

Preadmission testing (PAT) was first advocated in the early 1960s as a way to contain hospital costs. If diagnostic investigations and laboratory studies were done before a patient was hospitalized, his preoperative length of stay would be brief, resulting in lower hospital room and board charges per stay. The effectiveness of PAT programs was still in doubt, however, in the late 1960s and early 1970s.

Program evaluators found that preadmission testing was not done for several reasons. Many physicians avoided preadmission testing because they had difficulty changing their ordering habits, or they were unwilling to "penalize patients for a diagnostic error that would preclude coverage under the PAT program." Patients, too, were unwilling to have outpatient tests, especially when they had to make several visits to outpatient clinics and "travel and time were important factors" (Mebs and Brewer, 1971).

A 1972 analysis of preadmission testing in Pennsylvania hospitals concluded that the probability of lowering patients' preoperative stay to zero or one day depended on the hospital, not on the type of PAT program. The study reported that

coordination between the admissions and [operating room] areas, work scheduling in the ancillary departments, and medical practice [had] greater impact than [preadmission testing] on preop [length

54

of stay]. [Reduced preoperative length of stay therefore] will result from the overall efficiency of hospital operation and not the initiation of a preadmission testing program alone (Barbero et al., 1977).

The authors of an Iowa study concurred, pointing out that preadmission testing would not be successful unless there was coordination among members of the hospital team. The researchers reported: "The future of PAT as a means of freeing hospital beds seems to depend upon the willingness of the physicians and other paramedical personnel to be aware of and utilize the program..." (Mebs and Brewer, 1971).

The same conclusion was reached by faculty and students at the Medical College of Ohio, Toledo, after completing their cost containment program that focused on the effects of preadmission testing.

DESCRIPTION OF CURRICULUM

This experiment in teaching cost containment essentially involved several students working on a single project. Its *objective* was to let students discover the link between reimbursement policies and medical practices. The costs of alternative medical care practices appeared to vary widely, adversely affecting quality.

In 1977, MCO students conducted a study of cholecystectomy patients to determine whether preadmission testing would significantly alter the costs of care. They agreed on the criterion that preoperative preparation of cholecystectomy patients would require a maximum of one day. They decided that the patient should be hospitalized the day before surgery so that he would have nothing by mouth from midnight on and would be ready to receive an intravenous saline enema, preoperative medication, and preparation of the operative site on the morning of surgery. The patient should not have to be hospitalized for routine presurgical testing or a workup for gallbladder disease.

In their analysis, the students considered chest X ray, electrocardiogram, urinalysis, complete blood and platelet count, prothrombin time, partial thromboplastin time, blood type and crossmatch, blood urea nitrogen, and serum electrolyte and creatinine determinations as routine presurgical testing. As part of the workup for gallbladder disease, they included upper gastrointestinal series, single- and double-dose cholecystogram, IV cholecystogram, and liver scan.

The students selected the records of 40 patients with uncomplicated gallbladder disease who had an elective cholecystectomy during the preceding three years. They assessed the laboratory work that had been done for each patient, noting those tests done on an outpatient basis and those done during hospitalization. The students further examined all tests not considered part of routine presurgical testing of a gallbladder disease workup and judged, with the help of faculty preceptors, if any were required to have been done in the hospital.

The students found that none of the patients needed to be hospitalized for laboratory work. Nonetheless, all patients had had routine presurgical laboratory studies done after admission. Although patients did not have to be admitted for a gallbladder disease workup, 16 patients (40 percent) had diagnostic testing after they had been hospitalized. Twenty-four patients did have at least one test performed before admission: eight patients had an oral cholecystogram, seven had an oral cholecystogram and an upper GI series, and five had nonspecific gallbladder tests on an outpatient basis. Three other patients had an IV cholecystogram, and one had a liver scan and echogram before admission.

When the students looked at the preoperative length of stay, they found that only six patients had had the optimal preoperative stay of one day. They calculated that the average actual preoperative length of stay was 3.5 days. The 40 patients studied stayed a total of 139 preoperative days. Since the charge for a semi-private room on the surgical floor in 1977 was $139, total room and board costs were $19,321. If the patients had stayed the optimum of one preoperative day, the cost would have been $5,560. According to the students, with preadmission testing, patients would have stayed 99 fewer days and would not have had to pay room and board charges totaling $13,761.

To determine whether a brief preoperative length of stay might increase the risk of complication, the students calculated patients' complication rate by preoperative length of stay. The students learned that the complication rate for patients who stayed two preoperative days was 18 percent. The complication rate for patients who stayed three preoperative days was 22 percent. For patients who stayed four preoperative days, the complication rate was 25 percent. Even though the sample of patients who developed complications was small, the students' analysis suggested that reducing the number of preoperative days to one per patient would not have posed additional risks.

Since risks to the patient did not seem to be significant, the students wondered why the preoperative length of stay and consequent hospital charges were so high. They reasoned that excessive use of the hospital for diagnostic testing might be owing to the type of health insurance coverage available at the time. In 1977, standard health insurance policies covered inpatient but not outpatient diagnostic testing. The students also considered physicians' habits. They believed that physicians often admitted patients early without considering the possibility of outpatient testing. Finally, the students felt that physicians admitted patients a few days before surgery to prepare them psychologically for the operation.

The students concluded that money and hospital-bed time could be saved by establishing an optimal preoperative stay for a given surgical procedure. They did note, however, several problems with this approach. In the first place, it would probably be difficult to obtain physician compliance with such a plan. Medical authorities would not easily agree on the optimal number of preoperative days for all surgical procedures. Physicians also would find it hard to agree on which tests should be done on an outpatient basis and which should be done in the hospital.

Second, having tests done on an outpatient basis might decrease hospital revenues. Decreased hospital use for testing might result in higher charges for other services to offset the loss of revenues, or it might reduce the number of testing personnel in a hospital. On the other hand, if tests were done in the hospital outpatient department, hospital revenue and personnel might not be reduced, only transferred.

Third, testing done outside the hospital might affect the quality of medical education. With fewer hospital admissions for diagnostic testing, there would be fewer patients for interns and residents to work up for treatment.

The reluctance of the students to take a firm stand on the issue was only too apparent. However, despite the lack of agreement on a needed reimbursement policy, they clearly saw the linkage between the policy and the medical practices, their relationship to costs, and how they could be altered.

In a separate study of preadmission testing, faculty asked the students to analyze orders for laboratory tests on the first day of hospitalization to decide which tests could have been done before admission and which could have been postponed. Each student involved in the analysis examined the workups of four previously admitted patients. The workups had been done by other students during clerkships in internal medicine and pediatrics, and they included the patient's history, results of physical examination, list of the patient's problems, orders for diagnostic tests, and treatment plan.

To help the students in their review, the faculty prepared a questionnaire for overall evaluation of the workup and cost analysis (Figure 5.1). After assessing the workup, the students listed, on the cost-analysis questionnaire, the total number of tests that had been ordered

FIGURE 5.1. Audit Form.

Column(s)
  1–6 Patient Number
       (I) Assessment

7	A.	Logically Follows from History and Physical Information	0. No 1. Yes	☐
8	B.	Description of Alternate Possibilities	0. No 1. Yes	☐

      (II) Problem List

9	A.	First Problem: Health Maintenance Listed	0. No 1. Yes	☐
10	B.	Listing all Active Problems	0. No 1. Yes	☐
11	C.	"Incomplete Data Base" Listing (When Applicable)	0. No 1. Yes	☐
12	D.	Logical Problems Listed—Not Overly Restricted	0. No 1. Yes	☐

     (III) Plan of Study

13	A.	Numbered and Listed According to Problem List	0. No 1. Yes	☐
14	B.	Appropriate to Problem	0. No 1. Yes	☐

15 (IV) Auditor's Impression of Diagnostic Process   0. Inadequate   1. Adequate   ☐

(V) Plan of Management

16   A. Numbered and Listed According to Problem List   0. No   1. Yes   ☐

17   B. Appropriate to Problem   0. No   1. Yes   ☐

18 (VI) Auditor's Impression of Treatment Plans   0. Inadequate   1. Adequate   ☐

(VII) Plan of Patient Education

19   A. Numbered and Listed According to Problem List   0. No   1. Yes   ☐

20   B. Appropriate to Problem   0. No   1. Yes   ☐

21   C. Specific Information Given Patient and Family   0. No   1. Yes   ☐

22   D. Role of Patient and Family Specified   0. No   1. Yes   ☐

23 (VIII) Auditor's Impression of Education Plans   0. Inadequate   1. Adequate   ☐

24 (IX) Auditor's Impression about the Overall Medical Care Process as Documented at the Time of Initial Workup   1. Excellent   2. Above average   3. Average   4. Below average   ☐

25 (X) Expected Prognosis on the Basis of the Medical Care Process   1. Good   2. Poor   3. Indeterminate from available information   ☐

26–27 (XI) Cost Analysis: First Day's Orders
    A. Total Number of Tests Ordered   ☐☐

FIGURE 5.1. *(continued)*

28–32	B.	Total Cost of These Tests	☐☐☐☐☐
33–34	C.	Number of Minimum Necessary Tests Pertinent to the Problems of the Patient	☐☐
35–39	D.	Cost of Minimum Necessary Tests (Pertinent to the Problem of the Patient)	☐☐☐☐☐
40–41	E.	Number of Tests Which Could Have Been Delayed	☐☐
42–46	F.	Cost of Those Which Could Have Been Delayed	☐☐☐☐☐
47–48	G.	How Many Tests Could Have Been Performed Prior to This Elective Admission?	☐☐
49–53	H.	Cost of Tests That Could Have Been Performed Prior to This Elective Admission	☐☐☐☐☐
80	Card #	☐	

and the cost. They entered the minimum number of tests that were necessary, based on their evaluation of the patient's history, physical, and problem list. Next, the students determined the number and cost of the fewest essential tests that could have been postponed, as well as the number and cost of the tests that could have been done before admission.

The students evaluated a total of 262 patient workups and found that 2,943 tests had been ordered on the first day of hospitalization. They considered 2,440 (83 percent) of these tests necessary. Of the necessary tests, the students felt that 444 (18 percent) could have been postponed and 979 (40 percent) could have been done before admission (Table 5.1).

The charges for all hospital tests done on the day of admission were $40,272; the charges for necessary tests, however, were $34,150. The total cost of tests that could have been postponed was $4,402; for tests that could have been done before admission, the cost was $10,623 (Table 5.1).

On the day of admission, an average of 11 tests (costing $154) was ordered per patient. If only the minimum number of necessary tests had been performed, each patient, on the average, would have had two fewer tests and would have paid $24 less. In total, savings of about 10-20 percent could have been realized if only necessary tests had been done.

When the students broke down the findings by diagnostic categories, they learned that the largest discrepancy between the number of tests ordered and the number of necessary tests occurred among patients with endocrine diseases. For the 15 patients with endocrine problems, 299 tests were ordered, but only 218 (73 percent) were considered necessary. The total cost of all tests for these patients was $2,335; the cost of necessary tests was $1,751 (Table 5.2).

Through further analysis of the minimum of essential tests, the students discovered that 18 percent could have been postponed, generating a savings of $4,781 (Table 5.3). These figures averaged out to two

TABLE 5.1. **Summary Results of 262 Audits of Student Clerks by Their Peers During a Community Medicine Clerkship, 1976-77**

Category	Total	Average Per Patient
Number of patients evaluated	262	—
All tests ordered	2,943	11
Minimum necessary	2,440	9
Could have been done before admission	979	4
Could have been postponed	444	2
Charges for all tests ordered	$40,272	$154
Minimum necessary	34,150	130
Could have been done before admission	10,623	41
Could have been postponed	4,402	17

Reprinted with permission from: Garg, M.L., Gliebe, W.A., Kleinberg, W.M.: "Student Peer Review of Diagnostic Tests at the Medical College of Ohio." *Journal of Medical Education* 54 (1979): 852–854.

TABLE 5.2. Comparison of Tests Ordered by Student Clerks and Tests Judged by 68 Peers to be Minimum Necessary Plus Associated Charges by Diagnostic Categories, 1976–77

Diagnosis	No. of Patients	No. of Tests Ordered	No. (%) Minimum Necessary	Total Charges	Charges for Minimum (%)
Neoplasms	17	210	189 (90)	2,440	2,200 (91)
Endocrine	15	299	218 (73)	2,335	1,751 (75)
Circulatory	36	435	361 (83)	3,788	3,333 (88)
Digestive	7	100	93 (93)	1,192	1,144 (96)
Musculoskeletal	69	666	606 (91)	12,098	10,646 (88)
Congenital anomalies	17	154	134 (87)	2,823	2,682 (95)
Symptoms and ill-defined conditions	9	96	81 (84)	1,245	1,108 (89)
Miscellaneous	92	983	757 (77)	14,571	11,511 (79)
Total	262	2,943	2,443 (83)	40,462	33,875 (85)

Reprinted with permission from: Garg, M.L., Gliebe, W.A., Kleinberg, W.M.: "Student Peer Review of Diagnostic Tests at the Medical College of Ohio." *Journal of Medical Education* 54(1979): 852–854.

fewer tests and $17 less per patient. Although some of these tests might have had to be done at a later date, the students said, "It is likely that a substantial portion might not have been needed. Increased testing often leads to a large number of false positive tests and thus to a large number of secondary tests for follow-up" (Garg et al., 1979).

The students also found that 40 percent of the minimum necessary tests could have been done before admission. These tests accounted for 31 percent of the total cost of testing (Table 5.3). On the average, each patient could have had four tests done on an outpatient basis and could have saved $41 for this admission.

Preadmission testing would have saved $766 for patients with endocrine disorders, $935 for patients with circulatory problems, and $2,335 for patients with musculoskeletal problems (Table 5.3).

CONCLUSIONS

The analysis of preadmission testing had an objective beyond identifying the reimbursement, cost, and medical practices linkages. It placed students in the position of criticizing the judgment of practicing

TABLE 5.3. Percent of Tests Recommended by 58 Student Clerks to be Done before Admission and/or Postponed Plus Associated Charges by Diagnostic Categories, 1976–77

Diagnosis	No. of Patients	No. of Minimum Necessary Tests	No. (%) of Tests That Could Be		Total Charges for Minimum Necessary Tests	Charges (%) for Tests That Could Be	
			Done Before Admission	Postponed		Done Before Admission	Postponed
Neoplasms	17	190	70 (37)	19 (10)	2,027	811 (40)	203 (10)
Endocrine	15	217	59 (27)	67 (31)	1,740	766 (44)	574 (33)
Circulatory	36	362	101 (28)	51 (14)	3,340	935 (28)	367 (11)
Digestive	7	93	36 (39)	11 (12)	1,144	366 (32)	80 (7)
Musculoskeletal	69	603	223 (37)	114 (19)	10,615	2,335 (22)	1,274 (12)
Congenital anomalies	17	134	83 (62)	21 (16)	2,673	1,123 (42)	160 (6)
Symptoms and ill-defined conditions	9	81	39 (48)	18 (22)	1,112	345 (31)	167 (15)
Miscellaneous	92	760	365 (48)	144 (19)	11,499	3,910 (34)	1,610 (14)
Total	262	2,440	976 (40)	439 (18)	34,150	10,691 (31)	4,781 (14)

Adapted from: Garg, M.L., Gliebe, W.A., Kleinberg, W.M.: "Student Peer Review of Diagnostic Tests at the Medical College of Ohio." *Journal of Medical Education* 54(1979): 852–854.

physicians so they would learn not from a simulated patient and fictitious practitioner but from actual cases. Both exercises exposed students to cost control before they had formed a definitive conception of treatment behavior. They sought to contribute to cost-conscious behavior in future practice. Finally, they addressed the obligation of medical schools to define "acceptable standards for the utilization of tests and procedures" (Cooper, 1977). For the students, the audit made them realize that physicians are responsible for maintaining high standards of knowledge in clinical judgment to avoid unnecessary diagnostic searches, and that awareness of cost can influence physicians' decisions regarding hospitalization and diagnostic tests.

Preadmission testing is now an established standard and is included in most insurance programs. However, the critical evaluation of programs such as early discharge and home care can be carried out in a similar fashion.

REFERENCES

1. Barbero, Donna M., Shuman, L.J., and Swinkola, R.B. "An Evaluation of Various Presurgical Testing Procedures." *Inquiry* 14 (December 1977): 369–383.

2. Cooper, John A.D. "Medical Education: Past, Present and Future." *New England J. Med.* 297:17 (1977): 941–943.

3. Garg, Mohan L., Gliebe, W.A., and Kleinberg, W.M. "Student Peer Review of Diagnostic Tests at the Medical College of Ohio." *J. Medical Education* 54 (1979): 851–854.

4. Mebs, James E., and Brewer, John W. "Preadmission Testing." *Hospitals*, Jan. 16, 1971.

6   A New Clinico-Pathological Conference (CPC)

> The case presentation method is limited by its lack of attention to the techniques of clinical data collection and its tendency to deal with abstraction rather than with patients. A better approach is to have students first interview the patient briefly before the group.
> —George I. Engel

In 1900, Walter B. Cannon, while a student at Harvard, proposed a case method of teaching medicine based on that used to teach law students. Through what came to be known as the Clinico-Pathological Conference (CPC), Cannon hoped to correct some of the deficiencies in medical teaching by using a three-part system involving the presentation of an actual medical case history, study of the facts of the case, and discussion. He explained that students should study in detail the data in a patient's case history to arrive at a differential diagnosis of the patient's problem and the prognosis for the patient. Then, before issuing a formal plan of treatment, students should discuss the case with an instructor. Over the following decade, Drs. Cabot and Wright refined the case method of medical teaching. These studies are, of course, still published regularly in the *New England Journal of Medicine*.

Recent years have witnessed the active questioning by practitioners and by the *New England Journal of Medicine* itself of the continued use of the CPC. Revisions to include both social and clinical factors as the basis for treatment are reflected in the Clinico-Sociologic Conference published occasionally in the *American Journal of Medicine*. Such change and adaptation is a sign of the basic strength of the CPC as an educational tool. Since high quality, yet cost-effective, medical practice has become a predominant public issue, it seemed appropriate to utilize the CPC to perform yet another task in the education of contemporary physicians.

DESCRIPTION OF CURRICULUM

In 1977, the traditional CPC was modified at the Medical College of Ohio to include social and economic as well as clinical data in the process of patient management. The program was initiated in four of the ten body systems which then constituted the clinical science curriculum, beginning with the infectious-disease curriculum. The project was coordinated with the chairman of the college's infectious disease committee. Among the *objectives* of this program, the faculty sought to establish a systematic format for case presentation and to provide tools for assessing students' interpersonal relations with their patients and their data collection procedures. Most importantly, the program at the Medical College of Ohio was designed to emphasize cost-effective management of diagnosis and treatment, and to focus on the financial consequences of medical decision-making for the patient, his family, and society.

Two hours were allotted to replace one of the more traditional clinical conferences initially scheduled. A CPC on a case of meningitis was organized to include several components:

1. A general description along with subjective and objective findings on the day the patient was admitted to hospital (Figure 6.1)
2. A summary of the patient's progress during each hospital day (Figure 6.2)
3. A graphic presentation of the patient's treatment record (Figure 6.3)
4. A day-by-day list of all medical tests that had been ordered, the tests' results and their costs (Table 6.1)

The meningitis CPC differed from a traditional case presentation in two ways. In the first place, the Patient Progress Summary was designed to make students' assessments easier. Secondly, the CPC listed all diagnostic tests and procedures, the day on which they were ordered, and their actual charges. These changes were designed to help familiarize students with the process of relating patient management and assessment with the physician's workup, finding discrepancies in the treatment plan, and determining the cost-effectiveness and appropriateness of diagnostic tests and procedures. They gave students practice in applying a problem-oriented approach to patient management, critically analyzing each medical decision step, and ordering medical tests selectively.

FIGURE 6.1. Case 1.

Case Presentation for Clinico–Pathological Conference

Admission: Subjective —

J.K., a 4 1/2 year old boy, was well until five hours prior to admission when he was noted to be listless. Four hours prior to admission his parents noted that his temperature was 102°F which increased to 105°F despite sponging and aspirin suppositories. Two hours prior to admission his fever continued and he vomited four times. He was taken to the Emergency Room at the Medical College of Ohio where he was noted to have a temperature of 105.4°F, was mentally confused and extremely irritable. He was thought to have a stiff neck and was admitted with a diagnosis of possible meningitis.

Past history was unremarkable with the exception of recurrent episodes of otitis media in his second year of life for which he had tympanostomy tubes placed bilaterally at the age of 20 months. Following an eye infection at the age of one year, he was found to have absent lacrimal ducts.

Three weeks prior to this admission he was treated for bilateral otitis media with penicillin and appeared to recover uneventfully. His immunization series was reported to be adequate and included measles, mumps, and rubella vaccination. The family history is noncontributory. He has no known allergies, was currently taking no medications, and had normal developmental milestones.

Objective Findings:

Admission to the hospital, temperature was 105°F, pulse 120, respiratory rate 28, blood pressure 104/72; weight 18.14 kilograms, head circumference 51.5 cm. He was mentally confused, irritable and twitching. Horizontal nystagmus was noted but pupils were equal and reacted to light. Funduscopy revealed sharp discs and normal vessels. Ears were normal. He resisted neck flexion. There was no lymphadenopathy. No abnormalities were found in the chest, heart, or abdomen. Extremities revealed no deformities or tenderness. Skin revealed no rashes or bruises. Neurological examination revealed positive Brudzinski and Kernig signs, brisk knee jerks and negative Babinskis.

J.K. was admitted to the Intensive Care Unit and placed on cardiac monitoring, given phenobarbital, 50 mg every 8 hours, acetominophene, 200 mg every 4 hours and intravenous ampicillin, 1.5 gms every 4 hours with maintenance fluids.

FIGURE 6.2. Patient progress summary.

Day of Stay	Subjective Findings	Objective Findings	ASSESSMENT
			The following questions need to be answered in order to assess the progress of patient for each day for which subjective and objective findings have been given.
			(1) What is happening to the patient?
			(2) What is the problem?
			(3) What is likely cause or causes?
			(4) Is enough information available delineating problem and judging patient's course?
			(5) What, if any, other information or tests would you like to have? Specify.
			(6) Have too many tests been ordered? If yes, please specify.
			(7) Could less expensive and/or more reliable tests have been ordered? If yes, specify.
Day 1: Eight Hours After Admission.	J.K. complains of his back hurting. His mother remembered that he had been exposed to a 10 month old boy with primary tuberculosis.	Responsive, alert. No seizure activity. No neurologic deficits. Urine output 170 cc.	
Day 2:	J.K. complains of an earache.	Alert, talkative. TM's appear normal.	

Day 3:	J.K. wants to eat and go home.	Appears fine. Neck still stiff. Started on full liquids orally.
Day 5:	J.K. feels fine, eating well, sleeping well	
Day 9:	No complaints. His mother remembers that a cousin had infectious mononucleosis two months before.	(see graph) No neck stiffness. Tonsils erythematous, mildly enlarged. Palpable cervical nodes. I.V. sites not inflamed.
Day 10:	J.K. feels fine but is constipated.	Palpable liver edge.
Day 11:	Alert and not sick.	No organomegaly.
Day 13:	J.K. feels fine.	
Day 16:	J.K. feels fine.	P.E. essentially normal. PLAN: Discharged home. Continue on oral chloramphenicol 450 mg. Q.I.D. for 10 days. Begin FeSO$_4$ syrup 40 mg. Fe p.o. T.I.D. for 50 days. Return to clinic for follow-up in 4 days.

TABLE 6.1. Medical Tests, Their Results, and Their Costs

TEST	CHARGES	ADMISSION RESULT OF TEST ORDERED	IMPOR- TANCE*	DAY 1 RESULT OF TEST ORDERED	IMPOR- TANCE*	DAY 2 RESULT OF TEST ORDERED	IMPOR- TANCE*	DAY 3 RESULT OF TEST ORDERED	IMPOR- TANCE*
Hemogl/HCT	$ 4.00	11.8/37							
WBC × 10¹	2.50	9.9							
P S		70 11							
Diff. L M	3.50	17 2							
Platelets	4.00	Adeq.							
Retic Ct.	4.00			3.8					
Sed. Rate	4.00								
URINE									
Pro Glu				0 0		0 0			
Ke Bld				4+0		1+0			
Sp. Gr./pH	3.50	1.040		1.012/5		1.031/6			
Micro	–			(rare epith- elia cell)		0–3 WBC			
Na⁺ (per 24 hr)	4.00					71			
CSF									
Cell Ct RBC/WBC	4.50	1500/10,000				4698/4096			
Diff. P/L	3.50	95/5				94/6			
Prot./Blu	7.00	465/14				186/62			
LDH	5.00	76				158			
Gram Stain	4.00	Neg.							
AFB Stain	8.00	Neg.							
BLOOD									
Glu/BUN	3.00	138/16							
Creat.	4.50	0.7							
Na K		138 3.8				139 5		141 4.6	
Ele. Lytes Cl CO₂	14.00	104 20				104 20		107 20	

70

Ca^{++}		9.6			
Uric Acid	4.50			5.3	
Fe/TIBC	13.00	32/315			
Rheumatoid Factor	6.00				
Cold Agglut.	5.00				
Mono Spot	4.50				
Febrile Agglut.	10.00				
ANA	6.00				
MICROBIOLOGY					
NP	7.00	Neg.			
Throat	7.00	Neg.			
Blood	13.00	Neg.			
CSF	12.00	H. inf. Type F	Sensitive to Ampi.	Neg.	
Urine	9.00	Neg.	Neg.		
RADIOLOGY					
Chest	20.00				
Skull	31.00				
Mastoids	25.00				
Sinuses	21.00				
Brain Scan	75.00		ordered to be done next week		
Abd. Echogram	25.00				
Ga. Body Scan	100.00				
Skin Test PPD	2.00		Placed on forearm		
EEG	50.00				
Total # of Tests on a Given Day		21	5	11	1
Total Charge for a Given Day		$136.00	$81.50	$58.00	$14.00
Cumulative # of Tests to the Day		21	25	40	41
Cumulative Charges to the Day		$136.00	$217.50	$275.50	$289.50

TABLE 6.1. (continued)

TEST	CHARGES	DAY 4 RESULT OF TEST ORDERED	IMPOR- TANCE*	DAY 5 RESULT OF TEST ORDERED	IMPOR- TANCE*	DAY 6 RESULT OF TEST ORDERED	IMPOR- TANCE*	DAY 7 RESULT OF TEST ORDERED	IMPOR- TANCE*
Hemogl/HCT	$ 4.00			13		15.3		9/27	
WBC × 10³	2.50							10.8	
P S				56 3		56 1		70 0	
Diff. L M	3.50			29 7		36 6		29 1	
Platelets	4.00			Adequate		Incr.		Adequate	
Retic Ct.	4.00					Incr. RBC			
Sed. Rate								54	
URINE									
Pro Glu						02+			
Ke Bld						0.0			
Sp. Gr./pH	3.50	1.018		1.012		1.016/6			
Micro						0-1 WBC; 0-1RBC			
Na⁺ (per 24 hr)	4.00								
CSF									
Cell Ct RBC/WBC	4.50					13/20			
Diff. P/L	3.50					8/78			
Prot./Blu	7.00								
LDH	5.00					403			
Gram Stain	4.00					Neg.			
AFB Stain	8.00					Neg.			
BLOOD									
Glu/BUN	3.00					128			
Creat.	4.50								
Na K		139 4.3							

Test	Charge				
Ele. Lytes Cl CO_2	14.00	105 21			
Ca⁺⁺					
Uric Acid	4.50				
Fe/TIBC	13.00				
Rheumatoid Factor	6.00				33/300
Cold Agglut.	5.00				Neg.
Mono Spot	4.50			Neg.	
Febrile Agglut.	10.00			Neg.	
ANA	6.00				

MICROBIOLOGY

Test	Charge				
NP	7.00				
Throat	7.00			X6 Neg.	
Blood	13.00			Neg.	
CSF	12.00			Neg.	
Urine	9.00				

RADIOLOGY

Test	Charge				
Chest	20.00			Normal	
Skull	31.00			Normal	
Mastoids	25.00			Normal	
Sinuses	21.00				
Brain Scan	75.00				Normal
Abd. Echogram	25.00				Normal
Ga. Body Scan	100.00				
Skin Test PPD	2.00	Neg.			
EEG	50.00				Normal

Total # of Tests on a Given Day		3	4	21	10
Total Charge for a Given Day		$19.50	$13.50	$173.00	$186.00
Cumulative # of Tests to the Day		44	8	69	79
Cumulative Charges to the Day		$309.00	$322.50	$495.50	$681.50

73

TABLE 6.1. *(continued)*

TEST	CHARGES	DAY 12 RESULT OF TEST ORDERED	DAY 12 IMPOR-TANCE*	DAY 13 RESULT OF TEST ORDERED	DAY 13 IMPOR-TANCE*	DAY 14 RESULT OF TEST ORDERED	DAY 14 IMPOR-TANCE*	DAY 15 RESULT OF TEST ORDERED	DAY 15 IMPOR-TANCE*
Hemogl./HCT	$ 4.00					10.1/31			
WBC $\times 10^1$	2.50					6.2			
P S						40 0			
Diff. L M	3.50					53 3			
Platelets	4.00					Incr.			
Retic Ct.	4.00					7.9			
Sed. Rate		53							
URINE									
Pro Glu									
Ke· Bld									
Sp. Gr./pH	3.50								
Micro									
Na⁺ (per 24 hr)	4.00								
CSF									
Cell Ct RBC/WBC	4.50					24/4			
Diff. P/L	7.00					3/1			
Prot./Blu	5.00					15/54			
LDH						6			
Gram Stain	4.00								
AFB Stain	8.00								
BLOOD									
Glu/BUN	3.00								
Creat.	4.50								
Ele. Lytes Na K Cl CO₂	14.00								
Ca⁺⁺									
Uric Acid	4.50								

Fe/TIBC 13.00
Rheumatoid Factor 6.00 Neg.
Cold Agglut. 5.00
Mono Spot 4.50
Febrile Agglut. 10.00
ANA 6.00 Neg.

MICROBIOLOGY

NP 7.00
Throat 7.00
Blood 13.00 Neg.
CSF 12.00
Urine 9.00 Neg.

RADIOLOGY

Chest 20.00
Skull 31.00
Mastoids 25.00
Sinuses 21.00
Brain Scan 75.00
Abd. Echogram 25.00
Ga. Body Scan 100.00
Skin Test PPD 2.00
EEG 50.00

Total # of Tests on a Given Day	3	1	10
Total Charge for a Given Day	$16.00	$4.00	$50.00
Cumulative # of Tests to the Day	82	83	93
Cumulative Charges to the Day	$697.50	$701.50	$751.50

a"Normal lungs but heart slightly enlarged.
b"Multiple projections showing irregular reticular-sclerotic pattern noticed in both parietal bones compatible with hair-on-end pattern, most commonly found in congenital, hemolytic anemia, but also found uncommonly in congenital heart disease; hemangioma, which should be considered in the differential diagnosis."
*UN = Useful and Necessary
*UNN = Useful and Not Necessary
*NN = Not Useful and Not Necessary

FIGURE 6.3. Treatment schedule and temperature record.

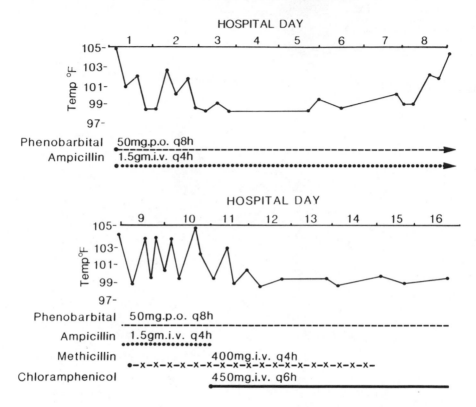

The chairman of the infectious disease committee selected five students from the class to present the case of meningitis. The presentations included:

1. Bacteriology of meningitis
2. Clinical and laboratory diagnosis of meningitis
3. Management of the disease
4. Outcome and prognosis for the patient
5. Cost-effectiveness of the patient's diagnosis and treatment

Each student worked with a faculty preceptor who helped him prepare his part of the presentation. Students met with their preceptors once a week, and a few days before the presentation all students and preceptors had a practice exercise to iron out any problems.

During the presentation, each student was allowed ten minutes to cover his topic and five minutes for limited discussion or questions from the class. Following the fifth presentation, an open discussion of all the issues related to meningitis took place.

A complete case protocol was sent to each member of the class one week before the CPC. Each student was asked to study the description of the case, the patient's progress, and the findings from medical tests to become familiar with the patient's problems. The students were asked to make their assessments of the patient's daily progress by completing the Patient Progress Summary (Figure 6.2).

Finally, the students were asked to decide the importance of each medical test. In the column labeled "Importance" on Table 6.1, the students indicated whether the test was appropriate. Using a code, they indicated if a test was useful and necessary (UN), useful but not necessary (UNN), or not useful and not necessary (NN) on the basis of the test's sensitivity, specificity and other treatment alternatives.

All five parts of the student presentation are important in themselves. However, the topic of discussion to which the Medical College of Ohio's case method of instruction has made a particular contribution is the cost-effectiveness of diagnosis and treatment. Again, as with other strategies, this one maintains the essential bridge between clinical experience and economic concerns.

The purpose of the presentation on cost-effectiveness was to examine the tests and the studies that had been done for the patient, and to use the case of meningitis as a framework for teaching students about quality assurance and cost containment. In addition, the presentation was designed to identify tests that could have been avoided without adding any risks to the patient's care or interfering with the diagnosis or evaluation of treatment. The exercise was meant to be critically instructive of the medical care that had been delivered in the case.

The student presenter analyzed the daily breakdown of medical tests (Table 6.1) and decided which were justified. He made the decision after looking at the laboratory tests and radiological studies that had been done during the patient's 16-day hospitalization and the treatment schedule, keeping in mind the tests and studies that increased the likelihood of reaching a diagnosis and posed no risk to the patient. The student's analysis reflected his reading in the literature and discussion with the preceptors.

When the presenter commented on the cost-effectiveness of prescribed medications, he noted that the least expensive drugs should have been used unless the patient's condition dictated otherwise. He concluded that the analysis of tests had shown him that fewer tests could have been ordered without subjecting the patient to unnecessary risks or compromising quality of medical care. It had also given him some idea of the costs of medical tests and made him think about the part that he could play in reducing health care costs while delivering optimum care.

The class evaluated the CPC exercise. The students' response to the modified CPC was positive, especially regarding the presentation of cost-effectiveness.

One of the later CPCs dealt with a patient with rheumatic fever and was presented during study of the cardiovascular body system. This CPC had the following objectives:

1. To reinforce students' recently acquired knowledge of cardiovascular physiology and pathology

2. To highlight the practical problems of diagnosis and treatment of rheumatic fever and its complications

3. To evaluate the cost-effectiveness of the treatment process

4. To allow students to question the patient (who was present) about her experience with the disease, adding a new dimension beyond the first CPC.

As in the case on meningitis, five students were selected to work with faculty preceptors and to prepare their discussion of the case itself, the etiology and pathophysiology of the disease, the epidemiology of rheumatic fever, the differential diagnosis, and the cost-effectiveness of the patient's care.

The student presenting the cost-effectiveness component met with clinical faculty members to discuss the specificity and sensitivity of each test and its appropriateness in managing the patient's problems. At the end of these discussions, the student placed each test into one of three categories, as before: useful and necessary (UN), useful but not necessary (UNN), or not useful and not necessary (NUNN). The student gave this information to a systems analyst who programmed the computer to print a display of the student's assessments and a summary of the costs of the tests. The printout also showed the number, percent, and total charges for the tests in each of the three categories (Tables 6.2, 6.3, 6.4).

TABLE 6.2. Cost-Benefit Analysis of Diagnostic Work-Up During First Hospitalization: Feb. 20 to April 3, 1973.

Test Report for: B.G.

TEST	CHARGE ($)	2/20 RESULT	2/21 RESULT	2/22 RESULT	2/23 RESULT	2/24 RESULT	2/25 RESULT	2/28 RESULT
LAB CBC	12.30	UN				NUNN		
Wh bld cnt								
Red bld cnt								
Hsb hct								
Differential								
Platelet cnt								
LAB SED RATE	6.20	UN				UN	NUNN	
LAB ASO TITER	14.20	UN						
LAB CRP LATEX QUAL	6.20	UN					UN	
LAB LE PREP	8.20		NUNN					
LAB ANTINUCL ANTIBOD	20.40						NUNN	
LAB VDRL	4.10						NUNN	
NCL T 3 TEST	10.70		NUNN				NUNN	
NCL T 4 TEST	15.00					NUNN		
LAB ELECTROLYTES	9.20		NUNN			NUNN		
LAB SALICYLATE	9.20							
LAB HVA	24.50							
LAB URINALYSIS	4.10							
Ph								
Spec grav								
Proteins								
Glucose								
Ketones								
Occult blood								
Microscopic								
LAB EMP FEC O/P/CULT	18.50	UN		NUNN		NUNN		
LAB PIN WORM TAPE	4.10	UN		NUNN		NUNN		
LAB EMP NORTH CULT	14.20	UN						
LAB BLOOD CULTURE	12.30						NUNN	
XR CHEST 1 VW	14.20		NUNN					
NCL HEART SCAN	60.00							
ELECTROCARDIOGRAM	14.80							
Daily Number of Tests:		8	5	2	2	5	4	1
Daily Charges:		$ 88.00	$ 66.60	$ 18.30	$ 78.50	$ 65.90	$ 47.00	$ 10.70
Cumulative Number of Tests:		8	13	15	17	22	26	27
Cumulative Charges		$ 88.00	$ 154.60	$ 172.90	$ 251.40	$ 317.30	$ 364.30	$ 375.00

79

TABLE 6.2. (continued)

Test Report for; B.G.

TEST	CHARGE ($)	3/2 RESULT	3/5 RESULT	3/7 RESULT	3/9 RESULT	3/12 RESULT	3/13 RESULT	3/16 RESULT
LAB CBC	12.30		NUNN		NUNN	NUNN		
Wh bld cnt								
Red bld cnt								
Hsb hct								
Differential								
Platelet cnt								
LAB SED RATE	6.20					NUNN		
LAB ASO TITER	14.20		UNN					
LAB CRP LATEX QUAL	6.20		NUNN					
LAB LE PREP	8.20							
LAB ANTINUCL ANTIBOD	20.40							
LAB VDRL	4.10							
NCL T 3 TEST	10.70			NUNN				
NCL T 4 TEST	15.00							NUNN
LAB ELECTROLYIES	24.80	NUNN						
LAB SALICYLATE	9.20	NUNN				NUNN	NUNN	NUNN
LAB HVA	24.50				UN	UN		
LAB URINALYSIS	4.10							
Ph								
Spec grav								
Proteins								
Glucose								
Ketones								
Occult blood								
Microscopic								
LAB EMP FEC O/P/CULT	18.50							
LAB PIN WORM TAPE	4.10							
LAB EMP NO&TH CULT	14.20							
LAB BLOOD CULTURE	12.30							
XR CHEST 1 VW	14.20							
NCL HEART SCAN	60.00							
ELECTROCARDIOGRAM	14.80						UNN	

		3/2	3/5	3/7	3/9	3/12	3/13	3/16
Daily Number of Tests:		2	3	1	2	4	2	2
Daily Charges:		$ 39.80	$ 24.70	$ 15.00	$ 21.50	$ 52.50	$ 24.00	$ 24.20
Cumulative Number of Tests:		29	32	33	35	39	41	43
Cumulative Charges		$ 414.80	$ 439.50	$ 454.50	$ 476.00	$ 528.50	$ 522.50	$ 576.70

80

Test Report for: B.G.

				DATE		
TEST	CHARGE ($)	3/20 RESULT	3/23 RESULT	3/24 RESULT	3/28 RESULT	4/3 RESULT
LAB CBC	12.30	NUNN				
Wh bld cnt						
Red bld cnt						
Hsb hct						
Differential						
Platelet cnt						
LAB SED RATE	6.20	NUNN				
LAB ASO TITER	14.20					
LAB CRP LATEX QUAL	6.20	NUNN				
LAB LE PREP	8.20					
LAB ANTINUCL ANTIBOD	20.40					
LAB VDRL	4.10					NUNN
NCL T 3 TEST	10.70					NUNN
NCL T 4 TEST	15.00					
LAB ELECTROLYTES	24.80					
LAB SALICYLATE	9.20	UN			UN	UN
LAB HVA	24.50		NUNN	NUNN		
LAB URINALYSIS	4.10					
Ph						
Spec grav						
Proteins						
Glucose						
Ketones						
Occult blood						
Microscopic						
LAB EMP FEC O/P/CULT	18.50					
LAB PIN WORM TAPE	4.10					
LAB EMP NO&TH CULT	14.20					
LAB BLOOD CULTURE	12.30					
XR CHEST 1 VW	14.20					
NCL HEART SCAN	60.00					
ELECTROCARDIOGRAM	14.80					

		3/20	3/23	3/24	3/28	4/3
Daily Number of Tests:		4		1	1	3
Daily Charges:		$ 33.90	$ 9.20	$ 9.20	$ 9.20	$ 34.90
Cumulative Number of Tests:		47	48	49	50	53
Cumulative Charges		$ 610.60	$ 619.80	$ 629.00	$ 638.20	$ 673.10

CLASSIFICATION	TESTS	PERCENT	CHARGES	PERCENT
TOTAL ALL TESTS	53	100.0	$ 673.10	100.0
I) Useful & Necessary	16	30.2	$ 164.90	24.5
II) Useful but Not Necessary	2	3.8	$ 21.00	3.1
III) Not Useful & Not Necessary	35	66.0	$ 487.20	72.4

81

TABLE 6.3. Cost-Benefit Analysis of Diagnostic Work-Up During Second Hospitalization: March 27 to June 19, 1974.

Test Report for: CASE, B.G.

TEST	CHARGE ($)	DATE 3/27 RESULT	3/29 RESULT	3/30 RESULT	3/31 RESULT	4/01 RESULT	4/02 RESULT	4/03 RESULT
LAB CBC	12.30	UN						
Wh bld cnt								
Red bld cnt								
Hsb hct								
Differential								
LAB SED RATE	6.20	UN						
LAB ASO TITER	14.20	UN						
LAB ANTINUCL ANTIBOD	20.40							
LAB CRP LATEX QUAL	6.20	UN	NUNN					
LAB ELECTROLYTES	24.80	UN						
LAB 12/60 BUN	7.10				NUNN	NUNN		
LAB SALICYLATE	9.20		UN	UN	UN	NUNN	NUNN	NUNN
LAB URINALYSIS	4.10	UN						
Ph								
Spec grav								
Proteins								
Glucose								
Ketones								
Occult blood								
Microscopic								
LAB EMP SORE TH CULT	7.10	UN						
LAB BLOOD CULTURE	12.30	UN						
XR CHEST 1 VW	14.20	UN	NUNN					NUNN
ELECTROCARDIOGRAM	14.80	UN	NUNN	NUNN				NUNN
Daily Number of Tests:		10	4	2	2	2	1	3
Daily Charges:		$ 116.20	$ 44.40	$ 24.00	$ 16.30	$ 16.30	$ 9.20	$ 38.20
Cumulative Number of Tests:		10	14	16	18	20	21	24
Cumulative Charges		$ 116.20	$ 160.60	$ 184.60	$ 200.90	$ 217.20	$ 226.40	$ 264.60

82

Test Report for; CASE, B.G.

DATE

TEST	CHARGE ($)	4/04 RESULT	4/05 RESULT	4/06 RESULT	4/07 RESULT	4/08 RESULT	4/09 RESULT	4/10 RESULT
LAB CBC	12.30							
Wh bld cnt								
Red bld cnt								
Hsb hct								
Differential								
LAB SED RATE	6.20	NUNN						NUNN
LAB ASO TITER	14.20	NUNN						NUNN
LAB ANTINUCL ANTIBOD	20.40							
LAB CRP LATEX QUAL	6.20						NUNN	
LAB ELECTROLYTES	24.80		NUNN					
LAB 12/60 BUN	7.10							
LAB SALICYLATE	9.20							
LAB URINALYSIS	4.10	NUNN	NUNN	NUNN	NUNN	UN	NUNN	UN
Ph								
Spec grav								
Proteins								
Glucose								
Ketones								
Occult blood								
Microscopic								
LAB EMP SORE TH CULT	7.10							
LAB BLOOD CULTURE	12.30							
XR CHEST 1 VW	14.20							
ELECTROCARDIOGRAM	14.80							

		4/04	4/05	4/06	4/07	4/08	4/09	4/10
Daily Number of Tests:			2	1	1	1	2	3
Daily Charges:		$ 20.60	$ 34.00	$ 9.20	$ 9.20	$ 9.20	$ 29.60	$ 29.60
Cumulative Number of Tests:		27	29	30	31	32	34	37
Cumulative Charges		$ 291.20	$ 328.20	$ 337.40	$ 346.60	$ 355.80	$ 385.40	$ 415.00

83

TABLE 6.3. (continued)

Test Report for; CASE, B.G.

TEST	CHARGE ($)	DATE 4/18 RESULT	4/22 RESULT	4/29 RESULT	5/08 RESULT	5/09 RESULT	5/16 RESULT	5/20 RESULT
LAB CBC	12.30					NUNN	NUNN	
Wh bld cnt								
Red bld cnt								
Hsb hct								
Differential								
Platelet cnt								
LAB SED RATE	6.20		NUNN	NUNN				
LAB ASO TITER	14.20		NUNN	NUNN				
LAB CRP LATEX QUAL	6.20			NUNN				
LAB ELECTROLYTES	24.80				NUNN			NUNN
LAB 12/60 BUN	7.10							
LAB SALICYLATE	9.20							
LAB URINALYSIS	4.10							
Ph						NUNN		
Spec grav								
Proteins								
Glucose								
Ketones								
Occult blood								
Microscopic								
LAB EMP NO&TH CULT	14.20					NUNN		
LAB BLOOD CULTURE	12.30					NUNN		
XR CHEST 1 VW	14.20	NUNN				NUNN		
ELECTROCARDIOGRAM	14.80	NUNN						
Daily Number of lests:		2	2	3	1	5	1	1
Daily Charges:		$ 29.00	$ 20.40	$ 26.60	$ 24.80	$ 57.10	$ 12.30	$ 24.80
Cumulative Number of Tests:		39	41	44	45	50	51	52
Cumulative Charges		$ 444.00	$ 464.40	$ 491.00	$ 515.80	$ 572.80	$ 585.20	$ 610.00

84

Test Report for; CASE, B.G.

DATE

TEST	CHARGE ($)	5/21 RESULT	5/25 RESULT	6/07 RESULT	6/19 RESULT
LAB CBC	12.30				
Wh bld cnt					
Red bld cnt					
Hsb hct					
Differential					
LAB SED RATE	6.20				
LAB ASO TITER	14.20				
LAB CRP LATEX QUAL	6.20				
LAB ELECTROLYTES	24.80	UN		NUNN	
LAB 12/60 BUN	7.10				
LAB SALICYLATE	9.20				
LAB URINALYSIS	4.10				
Ph					
Spec grav					
Proteins					
Glucose					
Ketones					
Occult blood					
Microscopic					
LAB EMP SORE TH CULT	7.10				
LAB BLOOD CULTURE	12.30			NUNN	
XR CHEST 1 VW	14.20			NUNN	
ELECTROCARDIOGRAM	14.80				

		5/21	5/25	6/07	6/19
Daily Number of Tests:		7	0	3	0
Daily Charges:		$ 9.20	$ 0.00	$ 38.20	$ 0.00
Cumulative Number of Tests:		53	53	56	56
Cumulative Charges		$ 619.20	$ 619.20	$ 657.40	$ 657.40

CLASSIFICATION	TESTS	PERCENT	CHARGES	PERCENT
TOTAL ALL TESTS	56	100.0	$ 657.40	100.0
I) Useful & Necessary	6	28.6	$ 171.40	26.1
II) Useful but Not Necessary	0	0.0	$ 0.00	0.0
III) Not Useful & Not Necessary	0	71.4	$ 486.00	73.9

TABLE 6.4. Cost-Benefit Analysis of Diagnostic Work-Up for Clinical Monitoring.

Test Report for; CASE, B.G.

TEST	CHARGE ($)	1/17/73 RESULT	2/01/73 RESULT	4/30/73 RESULT	6/14/73 RESULT	7/11/73 RESULT	9/25/73 RESULT	10/19/73 RESULT
LAB CBC	12.30	UN			NUNN	NUNN	NUNN	NUNN
LAB SED RATE	6.20	UN			NUNN	NUNN	NUNN	NUNN
LAB ASO TITER	14.20		UN		UN	UN	UN	UN
LAB CRP LATEX QUAL	6.20				NUNN	NUNN	NUNN	NUNN
LAB SICKLE SULVBILIT	4.50			NUNN				
LAB URINALYSIS	4.10	UN		NUNN	NUNN		NUNN	NUNN
LAB GLUCOSE	7.10	UN						
LAB EMP NO&TH CULT	14.20				NUNN			
XR CHEST 1 VW	14.20							
ELECTROCARDIOGRAM	14.80							
Daily Number of Tests:		5	1	2	6	5	6	6
Daily Charges:		$ 41.30	$ 4.50	$ 11.20	$ 57.20	$ 53.10	$ 57.20	$ 57.20
Cumulative Number of Tests:		5	6	8	14	19	25	31
Cumulative Charges:		$ 41.30	$ 45.80	$ 57.00	$ 114.20	$ 167.30	$ 224.50	$ 281.70

TEST	CHARGE ($)	11/19/73 RESULT	2/15/74 RESULT	8/20/74 RESULT	10/01/74 RESULT	1/09/75 RESULT	4/10/75 RESULT	8/11/77 RESULT
LAB CBC	12.30		NUNN	UN	NUNN			
LAB SED RATE	6.20		NUNN	UN				
LAB ASO TITER	14.20		UN	UN				
LAB CRP LATEX QUAL	6.20		NUNN					
LAB SICKLE SULVBILIT	4.50							
LAB URINALYSIS	4.10		NUNN	NUNN				
LAB GLUCOSE	7.10							
LAB EMP NO&TH CULT	14.20	NUNN	NUNN	UN	NUNN	NUNN		
XR CHEST 1 VW	14.20		NUNN					UN
ELECTROCARDIOGRAM	14.80		NUNN		NUNN			UN
Daily Number of Tests:		1	7	5	3	1	1	2
Daily Charges:		$ 14.20	$ 72.00	$ 51.00	$ 41.30	$ 14.20	$ 14.80	$ 29.00
Cumulative Number of Tests:		32	39	44	47	48	49	51
Cumulative Charges:		$ 295.90	$ 367.90	$ 418.90	$ 460.20	$ 474.40	$ 489.20	$ 518.20

CLASSIFICATION	TESTS	PERCENT	CHARGES	PERCENT
TOTAL ALL TESTS	51	100.0	$ 518.20	100.0
I) Useful & Necessary	17	33.3	$ 192.70	37.2
II) Useful but Not Necessary	0	0.0	$ 0.00	0.0
III) Not Useful & Not Necessary	34	66.7	$ 325.50	62.8

Before the conference, students received a copy of the case (Figure 6.4) and the day-by-day breakdown of the diagnostic tests and procedures ordered for the patients, their results and charges (Table 6.2, 6.3, 6.4). During the conference, the student who acted as coordinator of the presentation briefly reviewed the case with the class.

The first presenter gave an in-depth discussion of the etiology and pathophysiology of rheumatic fever using slides. He related the classical findings to the case. The student presenting the epidemiology of rheumatic fever emphasized the relationships between the occurrence of rheumatic fever and the family-social situation of the patient.

In the presentation on the differential diagnosis of the case, the student observed that the constitutional symptoms described for the patient (B.G.) at the beginning of her illness were nonspecific and could be attributed to a variety of conditions. He went on to analyze the decision processes used for diagnosis during the patient's two hospitalizations.

During the cost-effectiveness analysis of the case, the student pointed out:

In recent years the public, government, and private agencies have been concerned about the high cost of health care. One significant aspect of the cost issue revolves around laboratory testing. The question every good physician must ask him- or herself is: when is a test truly helpful in making a diagnosis? Physicians have been guilty of over-testing and this case is evidence of this fact.

If we examine the first five days of B.G.'s hospitalization we can evaluate the choices made by the physicians managing the case. We must not be too critical of the performance of the physician, considering hindsight is so much easier than foresight [and] many physicians are more aggressive when faced with a really sick child. Chiefly, we need to examine the main complaints and then utilize the physical findings and laboratory tests to make a diagnosis.

The patient's main complaints [were] poor appetite, profuse sweating, and [fatigue], all highly nonspecific symptoms. Her pulse rate was high for a child of her age; her blood pressure was 100/60/mm Hg. Positive physical findings were limited to the heart.

Although the list of conditions in the differential diagnosis is quite long, a careful selection of laboratory screening tests eliminates many causes of heart disease. A wide variety of screening tests were utilized in this case, and they may have been justified in an attempt to arrive at the diagnosis, initiate specific therapy, discharge the patient sooner, result in less inconvenience to the patient, better utilization of hospital space, and a lower cost per hospital stay.

During the first hospitalization a total of 53 tests were performed. [Some] tests were essential to the diagnosis of this case. The tests I believe are important on the first hospital day are a complete blood count, erythrocyte sedimentation rate, antistreptolysin O titer, C-reactive protein, urinalysis, nose and throat cultures, and a blood culture. Daily blood cultures might be useful to [rule out] subacute bacterial endocarditis, [and they] are justified in view of the high mortality rate of bacterial endocarditis.

The only test really useful during the prolonged hospital stay [is determination of the patient's] salicylate level once a week to monitor therapeutic efficacy. A salicylate level costs $9.20, and performing that test once a day accumulates costs rapidly. Following the erythrocyte sedimentation rate at regular, but less frequent, intervals allows for observation of the course of the illness and the patient's response to therapy.

Other tests, I think, may also have been useful. The LE prep, anti-nuclear antibody, T_3 and T_4, and serum electrolytes might have been ordered, and in view of the patient's background, occult blood and parasites should have been checked in the stool. A chest X ray, electrocardiogram, and blood urea nitrogen may have been useful also.

However, [some] tests did not aid in the diagnosis or management of the case. Serology for syphilis and hepatitis-associated antigen [done] on the second hospital day were probably superfluous. The hematocrit, repeat ova and parasite tests probably were unnecessary. Pinworm tests already had been reported as positive. Many of the routine screening tests such as T_3 and DNA that were performed on the fifth, sixth, or seventh hospital day after a presumptive diagnosis of rheumatic fever were wholly unnecessary.

The medications used in the treatment of rheumatic fever are relatively inexpensive. One hundred aspirin tablets cost approximately $1.00; 100 tablets of penicillin cost approximately $2.40. Under the present circumstances, we are, therefore, more concerned about the side effects of the medications than their actual costs.

Nevertheless, if we include the hospital bed costs in addition to [the patient's] medications and laboratory tests, her first hospitalization cost almost $3,000. The cost incurred by the patient during the second hospitalization was twice as much as the first one. Moreover, the cost and strain on the child's family, lost educational opportunities, and long-term health-surveillance demands on the visiting nurse cannot be measured easily in dollars and cents. For B.G., *rheumatic fever is a disease that has monetary costs as well as social and physical costs.*

FIGURE 6.4. Case 2.

Case Presentation for Clinico-Socio-Economic Conference

B.G. (birthdate June 26, 1965) is a black girl who was seen in the Pediatric Clinic at the Medical College of Ohio for the first time on January 17, 1973, on referral from the school health nurse because of a poor appetite, sweating a great deal, and tiring easily. The family had moved to Toledo eleven months previously and the patient's mother reported that she had had no serious illnesses or hospitalization. She had had no tonsillitis or sore throats in the previous year. She was afebrile, had a pulse of 130 per minute, blood pressure of 100/60, respiratory rate of 20, a height of 51 inches and a weight of 49½ pounds. Positive physical findings were limited to her heart, and revealed a systolic thrill at the left sternal border and a Grade IV/VI pansystolic murmur at the apex and left sternal border. Laboratory findings are on the flow sheet. She was referred to the Pediatric Cardiology Clinic where she was seen one month later and admitted to the Pediatric Ward.

Further history upon admission revealed no history of migratory joint pains or rash; no significant fevers; no edema, syncope, orthopnea, or paroxysmal nocturnal dyspnea. Her mother related that their family doctor in Georgia had made no mention of a heart murmur. Her mother thought that the child may have worms. Her mother and brother had sickle cell trait. There was no history of heart disease, diabetes mellitus, nerve problems, or epilepsy in the family. The mother lived alone with her three children and was supported by ADC. The child was then in the first grade and had repeated that grade for reasons unknown to the mother. Pulse rate was 144, blood pressure 100/74, weight 46 pounds, and height 50½ inches. She was afebrile. Physical exam revealed an alert, thin, seven year old black girl in no acute distress. Positive physical findings were again limited to the heart which demonstrated a regular rhythm and tachycardia, a prominent precordial heave, and an apical thrill. There was a Grade IV/VI systolic murmur, heard best at the apex with a gallop rhythm.

The patient remained comfortable and in no distress. She was begun on treatment with penicillin and prednisone on the second hospital day and digoxin on the third hospital day. The pulse rate came down to 100 by the fourth hospital day and remained 80–110 throughout her hospital course. Her condition remained stable on bed rest and she was discharged on April 4, 1973, on moderate restriction of activity, on aspirin which had begun on the twentieth hospital day, and penicillin G tablets to be taken daily at home. She was to return for regular follow-up in the Rheumatic Fever Clinic.

FIGURE 6.4. (*continued*)

The child kept her monthly appointments in the Rheumatic Fever Clinic, was restarted on digoxin one month after discharge, and was given monthly injections of Benzathine penicillin. Regular appointments were kept until January, 1974. Contact was lost until March 27, 1974, when she was seen in the Emergency Room at the Medical College of Ohio with a pulse rate of 140, respiratory rate of 30, a gallop rhythm, and a liver palpable 2 cm. below the right costal margin.

On admission to the hospital on March 27, 1974, she had a height of 52¾ inches, a weight of 56½ pounds, temperature of 100.4° F, pulse of 140, and a respiratory rate of 30. She was not in distress and positive physical findings were again limited to her heart. The precordium was very active with an apical beat located in the fifth left intercostal space 1 cm. lateral to the mid-clavicular line; there was a precordial heave and a tapping character on palpation; S_1 was loud and snappy in character and S_2 was soft and appeared to be physiologically split. A holosystolic murmur was heard at the apex, radiating to the back and to the axilla; it was Graded at III-IV/VI. There was also a mid-diastolic murmur heard at the apex. Laboratory studies were obtained as reported on the flow sheet. She was begun on Penicillin G intravenously (for ten days), on digoxin on the first hospital day, aspirin on the second hospital day, and prednisone on the seventh hospital day. She appeared comfortable on bed rest and pulse rate came down to 100 by the fifth hospital day and remained between 80 and 120 subsequently throughout her hospitalization. On severe activity restriction and bed rest she remained comfortable, afebrile, asymptomatic, and gained weight progressively without evidence of edema. After ten days, the child was started on monthly intra-muscular Benzathine, Penicillin G. She was discharged after three months and continued on aspirin and digoxin to be followed up in the Rheumatic Fever Clinic with monthly injections of Benzathine penicillin.

Appointments were kept regularly with the assistance of the Community Nursing Service, and the frequency of follow-up visits was reduced to every three months with the Visiting Nurse providing monthly injections of Benzathine penicillin in the home. The child missed three consecutive appointments in 1976 and did not return for reevaluation until January 1977 when her condition appeared to be stable. She missed her appointment in July of 1977 but after Community Nursing Services was contacted she was seen in August of 1977 when again her condition was stable. She missed her appointment on February 23, 1978. Community Nursing Services continues to visit the home every 28 days to provide her with home reassessment and her monthly Benzathine penicillin injections.

TABLE 6.5. Diagnostic Work-Up During First Hospitalization: Feb. 20 to April 3, 1973.

Test Report for; B.G.

TEST	CHARGE ($)	2/20 RESULT	2/21 RESULT	2/22 RESULT	2/23 RESULT	2/24 RESULT	2/25 RESULT	2/28 RESULT
LAB CBC	12.30							
Wh bld cnt		9.4						
Red bld cnt		4.12						
Hsb hct		11.2/34				/36		
Differential		70/28/1/0						
Platelet cnt		ADEQUATE						
LAB SED RATE	6.20	48/40				25/22	23	
LAB ASO TITER	14.20	125						
LAB CRP LATEX QUAL	6.20	1:5					POS.UNDILUTE	
LAB LE PREP	8.20		NEGATIVE					
LAB ANTINUCL ANTIBOD	20.40						1:8	
LAB VDRL	4.10		NEGATIVE					30.4%
NCL T 3 TEST	10.70		7.7					
NCL T 4 TEST	15.00							
LAB ELECTROLYTES	24.50					136/4./97/25		
LAB SALICYLATE	9.20							
LAB HVA	24.50		NEGATIVE					
LAB URINALYSIS	4.10							
Ph		6						
Spec grav		1.017						
Proteins		TR						
Glucose		0						
Ketones		0						
Occult blood		0						
Microscopic		RARE WBC						
LAB EMP FEC O/P/CULT	18.50	NEGATIVE		POSITIVE	NEGATIVE	NEGATIVE		
LAB PIN WORM TAPE	4.10			NO B-STREP		NEGATIVE		
LAB EMP NO&TH CULT	14.20	B-ST.GP.14EH						
LAB BLOOD CULTURE	12.30	NEG AT 48HRS						
XR CHEST 1 VW	14.20		WNI		ELG-LT.R&LVT			
NCL HEART SCAN	60.00						MIN CARD IMP	
ELECTROCARDIOGRAM	14.80							
Daily Number of Tests:		8	5	2	2	5	4	1
Daily Charges:		$ 88.00	$ 66.60	$ 18.30	$ 78.50	$ 65.90	$ 47.00	$ 10.70
Cumulative Number of Tests:		8	13	15	17	22	26	27
Cumulative Charges		$ 88.00	$154.60	$172.90	$251.40	$317.30	$364.30	$375.00

91

TABLE 6.5. (*continued*)

Test Report for; B.G.

TEST	CHARGE ($)	DATE 3/2 RESULT	3/5 RESULT	3/7 RESULT	3/9 RESULT	3/12 RESULT	3/13 RESULT	3/16 RESULT
LAB CBC	12.30							
Wh bld cnt			17.4			16.8		
Red bld cnt			4.22			4.3		
Hsb hct			11.9/37		12.2/38	12.2/37		
Differential			70/28/1/0			60/33/7/0		
Platelet cnt			ADEQUATE			7/6		
LAB SED RATE	6.20		8					
LAB ASO TITER	14.20							
LAB CRP LATEX QUAL	6.20		NEGATIVE					
LAB LE PREP	8.20							
LAB ANTINUCL ANTIBOD	20.40							
LAB VDRL	4.10							
NCL T 3 TEST	10.70							
NCL T 4 TEST	15.00	6.5		7.3				
LAB ELECTROLYTES	24.80	136/4./96/22				148/5/110/28		
LAB SALICYLATE	9.20				56	29	38.7	31.4
LAB HVA	24.20							
LAB URINALYSIS	4.10							
Ph								
Spec grav								
Proteins								
Glucose								
Ketones								
Occult blood								
Microscopic								
LAB EMP FEC O/P/CULT	18.50							
LAB PIN WORM TAPE	4.10							
LAB EMP NO&TH CULT	14.20							
LAB BLOOD CULTURE	12.30							
XR CHEST 1 VW	14.20							
NCL HEART SCAN	60.00							
ELECTROCARDIOGRAM	14.80						DIGITALIS EF	
Daily Number of Tests:		2	3	1	2	4	2	2
Daily Charges:		$ 39.80	$ 24.70	$ 15.00	$ 21.50	$ 52.50	$ 24.00	$ 24.20
Cumulative Number of Tests:		29	32	33	35	39	41	43
Cumulative Charges		$414.80	$439.50	$454.50	$476.00	$528.50	$552.50	$576.70

92

Test Report for; B.G.

				DATE		
TEST	CHARGE ($)	3/20 RESULT	3/23 RESULT	3/24 RESULT	3/28 RESULT	4/3 RESULT
LAB CBC	12.30					
Wh bld cnt		6.9				
Red bld cnt		3.94				
Hsb hct		10.8/34				
Differential		41/5T/3/4				
Platelet cnt		OK				
LAB SED RATE	6.20	12/8				
LAB ASO TITER	14.20					
LAB CRP LATEX QUAL	6.20					
LAB LE PREP	8.20					
LAB ANTINUCL ANTIBOD	20.40	NEGA-IVE				
LAB VDRL	4.10					
NCL T 3 TEST	10.70					31.9
NCL T 4 TEST	15.00					3/3
LAB ELECTROLYTES	24.80					
LAB SALICYLATE	9.20	25	27.1	30.0	24.0	18.0
LAB HVA	24.20					
LAB URINALYSIS	4.10					
Ph						
Spec grav						
Proteins						
Glucose						
Ketones						
Occult blood						
Microscopic						
LAB EMP FEC O/P/CULT	18.50					
LAB PIN WORM TAPE	4.10					
LAB EMP NO&TH CULT	14.20					
LAB BLOOD CULTURE	12.30					
XR CHEST 1 VW	14.20					
NCL HEART SCAN	60.00					
ELECTROCARDIOGRAM	14.80					
Daily Number of Tests:		4	1	1	1	3
Daily Charges:		$ 33.90	$ 9.20	$ 9.20	$ 9.20	$ 34.90
Cumulative Number of Tests:		47	48	49	50	53
Cumulative Charges		=610.60	$619.80	$629.00	$638.20	$673.10

93

TABLE 6.6. Diagnostic Work-Up During Second Hospitalization: March 27 to June 19, 1974.

Test Report for; CASE, B.G.

TEST	CHARGE ($)	3/27 RESULT	3/29 RESULT	3/30 RESULT	3/31 RESULT	4/01 RESULT	4/02 RESULT	4/03 RESULT
LAB CBC	12.30							
Wh bld cnt		9.2						
Red bld cnt		3.56						
Hsb hct		10.4/30						
Differential		77/18/3/2						
LAB SED RATE	6.20	51						
LAB ASO TITER	14.20	1:240						
LAB ANTINUCL ANTIBOD	20.40		1:50					
LAB CRP LATEX QUAL	6.20	1:50						
LAB ELECTROLYTES	24.80	191/4/108/23						
LAB 12/60 BUN	7.10				55.8	48.7		
LAB SALICYLATE	9.20		13.6	30.4	46.9	38.2	45.6	48.0
LAB URINALYSIS	4.10							
Ph		6						
Spec grav		1.009						
Proteins		0						
Glucose		0						
Ketones		0						
Occult blood		0						
Microscopic		8-10 WBC						
LAB EMP SORE TH CULT	7.10	NEG AT 48HRS						
LAB BLOOD CULTURE	12.30	X6 NEG 48HRS						
XR CHEST 1 VW	14.20	L ATR&VT ELG	UNCHANGED					CRDMG/CNGEST
ELECTROCARDIOGRAM	14.80	DIG. EFF LVH	DIG. EFF LVH	DIG. EFF LVH				DIG. EFF LVH
Daily Number of Tests:		10	4	2	2	2	1	3
Daily Charges:		$116.20	$ 44.40	$ 24.00	$ 16.30	$ 16.30	$ 9.20	$ 38.20
Cumulative Number of Tests:		10	14	16	18	20	21	24
Cumulative Charges		$116.20	$160.60	$184.60	$200.90	$217.20	$226.40	$264.60

94

Test Report for; CASE, B.G.

TEST	CHARGE ($)	4/4 RESULT	4/5 RESULT	4/6 RESULT	4/7 RESULT	4/8 RESULT	4/9 RESULT	4/10 RESULT
LAB CBC	12.30							
Wh bld cnt								
Red bld cnt								
Hsb hct								
Differential								
LAB SED RATE	6.20	79						15
LAB ASO TITER	14.20	1:340						1:240
LAB ANTINUCL ANTIBOD	20.40						20/256	
LAB CRP LATEX QUAL	6.20							
LAB ELECTROLYTES	24.80		137/5/99/27					
LAB 12/60 BUN	7.10							
LAB SALICYLATE	9.20	38.7	35.8	20.3	32.9	24.0	21.2	16.5
LAB URINALYSIS	4.10							
Ph								
Spec grav								
Proteins								
Glucose								
Ketones								
Occult blood								
Microscopic								
LAB EMP SORE TH CULT	7.10							
LAB BLOOD CULTURE	12.30							
XR CHEST 1 VW	14.20							
ELECTROCARDIOGRAM	14.80							

		4/4	4/5	4/6	4/7	4/8	4/9	4/10
Daily Number of Tests:		3	2	1	1	1	2	3
Daily Charges:		$ 29.60	$ 34.00	$ 9.20	$ 9.20	$ 9.20	$ 29.60	$ 29.60
Cumulative Number of Tests:		27	29	30	31	32	34	37
Cumulative Charges		$294.20	$328.20	$337.40	$346.60	$355.80	$385.40	$415.00

DATE

95

TABLE 6.6. (continued)

Test Report for; CASE, B.G.

TEST	CHARGE ($)	4/18 RESULT	4/22 RESULT	4/29 RESULT	5/8 RESULT	5/9 RESULT	5/16 RESULT	5/20 RESULT
LAB CBC	12.30							
Wh bld cnt						12.7	12.8	
Red bld cnt						4.05	4.41	
Hsb hct						12/39	13.1/41	
Differential						73/22/4/1	75/23/1/1	
Platelet cnt						OK	OK	
LAB SED RATE	6.20		2	2				15
LAB ASO TITER	14.20		1:240	1:170				
LAB CRP LATEX QUAL	6.20			NEGATIVE				
LAB ELECTROLYTES	24.80				140/4/104/23		·	143/3/104/23
LAB URINALYSIS	4.10							
Ph						2.5		
Spec grav						1.019		
Proteins						0		
Glucose						0		
Ketones						0		
Occult blood						0		
Microscopic						OK		
LAB EMP NO&TH CULT	14.20					NEG AT 48HRS		
LAB BLOOD CULTURE	12.30					X2 NEG 48 HRS		
XR CHEST 1 VW	14.20	L ATR&VT ELG				UNCHANGED		
ELECTROCARDIOGRAM	14.80	LVH,L DIG EF						
Daily Number of Tests:		2	2	3	1	5	1	1
Daily Charges:		$ 29.00	$ 20.40	$ 26.60	$ 24.80	$ 57.10	$ 12.30	$ 24.80
Cumulative Number of Tests:		39	41	44	45	50	51	52
Cumulative Charges		$444.00	$464.40	$491.00	$515.80	$572.90	$585.20	$610.00

Test Report for; CASE, B.G.

DATE

TEST	CHARGE ($)	5/21 RESULT	5/25 RESULT	6/7 RESULT	6/19 RESULT
LAB CBC	12.30				
Wh bld cnt					
Red bld cnt					
Hsb hct					
Differential					
LAB SED RATE	6.20				
LAB ASO TITER	14.20				
LAB CRP LATEX QUAL	6.20				
LAB ELECTROLYTES	24.80				
LAB 12/60 BUN	7.10				
LAB SALICYLATE	9.20			2.8	
LAB URINALYSIS	4.10	23			
Ph					
Spec grav					
Proteins					
Glucose					
Ketones					
Occult blood					
Microscopic					
LAB EMP SORE TH CULT	7.10				
LAB BLOOD CULTURE	12.30				
XR CHEST 1 VW	14.20			UNCHANGED	
ELECTROCARDIOGRAM	14.80			LVH,DIG,EFF	

		5/21	5/25	6/7	6/19
Daily Number of Tests:		1	0	3	0
Daily Charges:		$ 9.20	$ 0.00	$ 38.20	$ 0.00
Cumulative Number of Tests:		53	53	56	56
Cumulative Charges		$619.20	$619.20	$657.40	$657.40

97

TABLE 6.7. Diagnostic Work-Up for Clinical Monitoring.

Test Report for; CASE, B.G.

TEST	CHARGE ($)	1/17/73 RESULT	2/01/73 RESULT	4/30/73 RESULT	6/14/73 RESULT	7/17/73 RESULT	9/25/73 RESULT	10/19/73 RESULT
LAB CBC	12.30	NORMAL			NORMAL	NORMAL	NORMAL	NORMAL
LAB SED RATE	6.20	51			6	7	10	6
LAB ASO TITER	14.20				50	50	12	12
LAB CRP LATEX QUAL	6.20				NEGATIVE	NEGATIVE	NEGATIVE	NEGATIVE
LAB SICKLE SULVBILIT	4.50	POSITIVE (+)	HB ELECT AS					
LAB URINALYSIS	4.50	NORMAL		NORMAL	NORMAL		NORMAL	NORMAL
LAB GLUCOSE	7.10			102/127				
LAB EMP NO&TH CULT	14.20	NEGATIVE				NEGATIVE	NEGATIVE	NEGATIVE
XR CHEST 1 VW	14.20							
ELECTROCARDIOGRAM	14.80				CROMEGAL–LVH			
Daily Number of Tests:		5	1	2	6	5	6	6
Daily Charges:		$ 41.30	$ 4.50	$ 11.20	$ 57.20	$ 53.10	$ 57.20	$ 57.20
Cumulative Number of Tests:		5	6	8	14	19	25	31
Cumulative Charges:		$ 41.30	$ 45.80	$ 57.00	$ 114.20	$ 167.30	$ 224.50	$ 281.70

98

Test Report for; CASE, B.G.

DATE

TEST	CHARGE ($)	11/19/73 RESULT	1/15/74 RESULT	8/20/74 RESULT	10/01/74 RESULT	1/09/75 RESULT	4/10/75 RESULT	8/11/77 RESULT
LAB CBC	12.30		NORMAL	NORMAL	NORMAL			
LAB SED RATE	6.20		5	9	6			
LAB ASO TITER	14.20		50	120				
LAB CRP LATEX QUAL	6.20		NEGATIVE					
LAB SICKLE SULVBILIT	4.50							
LAB URINALYSIS	4.10		NORMAL	NORMAL				
LAB GLUCOSE	7.10							
LAB EMP NO&TH CULT	14.20	NEGATIVE	NEGATIVE	GPA, B-STREP				
XR CHEST 1 VW	14.20				LAH, LVH			
ELECTROCARDIOGRAM	14.80		LVH		LVH DIG.EFF	CARDIOMEGALY	LVH DIG.EFF	NO CHANGE LVH

		11/19/73	1/15/74	8/20/74	10/01/74	1/09/75	4/10/75	8/11/77
Daily Number of Tests:		1	7	5	3	1	1	2
Daily Charges:		$ 4.20	$ 72.00	$ 51.00	$ 41.30	$ 14.20	$ 14.80	$ 29.00
Cumulative Number of Tests:		32	39	44	47	48	49	51
Cumulative Charges:		$ 255.90	$ 367.90	$ 418.90	$ 460.20	$ 474.40	$ 489.20	$ 518.20

99

After the final student presentation, the patient, her mother, and the child's cardiologist were brought into the classroom, introduced and interviewed.

The cardiologist told the class:

I saw B.G. for the first time after [her] second hospitalization. Into the outpatient clinic came a chronically sick-looking, skinny little kid. You get a good feeling if you see patients improving. However, by our preventive medicine model, rheumatic fever should not even occur if strep infections could be controlled or eliminated. After the fact, there is no question that rheumatic fever can be a costly disease and B.G.'s hospital bills reflect that fact. Within the hospital bill were many costs that could have been eliminated and should not have been incurred and her relapse should not have occurred if proper planning and good compliance were carried out.

"It was terrible," Mrs. G. said when asked about B.G.'s illness.

I thought we weren't going to make it, but we made it and that's what is important. [B.G.] was a problem because she couldn't go up and down stairs. She either had to stay upstairs or stay downstairs. She was pretty sick. But she doesn't have a problem now. She can run and play and I make sure she [gets] her penicillin shot every month.

"I feel wonderful," said B.G.:

I can play for the Junior High basketball team. My heart doesn't give me any more trouble, and I can do everything the other kids do. They can play jump rope; I can, too. They wanted to put me back in the sixth grade this year but they didn't. I went to the seventh grade.

However, B.G's cardiologist pointed out:

[Her] school problem is a chronic one. All of those months of school she missed when in the hospital were critical. Initially, after her hospitalization she was required to have some instruction. From a cost accounting standpoint, we must consider the cost of a daily home tutor and the cost of repeating a school year.

Another aspect of B.G.'s medical treatment that should be considered is the cost to the parent and child of frequent clinic visits. "Here we have a mother and daughter who have to take three buses to get to the medical center," said the cardiologist.

> The child is too sick to really walk very long and then you have to wait to get the connecting bus. There isn't enough money to pay for cab fare either. Sometimes at the clinic, they have to wait, which is tiring. And finally, do you know what you have to do after you come on three buses? You have to go home on three more buses.
>
> A temporary solution is to have the public health nurse visit B.G. at home and give her the injections there. Having the visiting nurse go to the home [is] more reliable than having the patient come to the doctor's office or the clinic for her monthly injection. I might also add that B.G. has had enough cardiac involvement; she could ill afford another bout of rheumatic fever.

CONCLUSIONS

Class response to the Clinico-Pathologic Conference on rheumatic fever was favorable. The five student presenters said they gained experience in the preparation, organization, and delivery of medical information and in the formal analysis of medical care and economics. Other students said that the case presentation made previous lectures and readings on rheumatic fever fall into place. They felt that they had gained an appreciation for comprehensive health care, preventive medicine, and the social and monetary cost of the disease. No other case presentation in the curriculum, the students said, provided as much opportunity for learning or had greater personal impact.

The students remarked that through the case they became aware of the impact of cardiovascular disease on the patient. They had a greater understanding of the importance of judicious, logical, cost-conscious medical decision-making to meet the specific needs of patients and their families.

The modified case method has addressed some of the human and socioeconomic aspects of health care by scheduling interviews with patients and their families and assessing the personal and socioeconomic questions students ask in these interviews. It has increased students' awareness of cost by looking at the necessity of each test and at less expensive but equally effective drugs. It has spurred students to keep careful and systematic records of their objective and subjective findings and observations, as well as the logical pathways of decision-making.

The widespread applicability of this educational strategy should make it particularly effective at all levels of medical education. It can be adapted as part of medical grand rounds, as an independent CME program, or to undergraduates as described here. Further, it can be presented alone or in conjunction with other strategies or modules. Its flexibility makes it a potentially widespread option whose linkage of clinical practice and economic considerations is direct and logical. With experience, the additional effort required beyond current educational programming is minimal.

RESOURCE REQUIREMENTS FOR CPC CURRICULUM

1. Faculty

   a. At least two physicians, one working with the overall CPC curriculum, another serving as appropriate specialty clinical preceptor. Other physicians with clinically relevant specialties should be available as discussants.
   b. At least one member should specialize in health economics and cost-effective clinical decision-making analysis.
   c. Cooperation of faculty curriculum committees in allocating two hour time periods for such CPCs. One-fourth (25 percent) of all CPCs to incorporate cost-effectiveness would be a second year goal.
   d. Other staff to prepare student surveys and tabulate results would also be beneficial, although not essential.

2. Materials

   a. Cooperation of medical records department to permit presenting students access to case data.
   b. Outline of materials (as described here and attached) should be available to all students seven days before being presented.
   c. Appropriate visual presentation equipment for slides or videotapes.

3. Time

a. Two hours per CPC.
b. If 25 percent is goal as above, two or more CPCs per month would be required.
c. Meetings with curriculum committees are also essential.

4. Number of Students and Space

a. Lecture hall with audio-visual capability would be most desirable.
b. Any size group from 20 to an entire class can be effective.

5. Evaluation

a. Evaluations are completed by students before leaving the session, using Likert response categories.
b. Other vehicles should include relevant questions on examinations in that course.
c. Informal evaluations can also be made by clinical faculty as students begin clinical experiences.
d. Such CPCs can be continued during clerkship and residency training to reinforce desired objectives.
e. Long-term evaluation could include cost-effectiveness of student clinical practices during later clinical (residency) training.

6. Locus in Curriculum

This program can be presented almost anywhere in the medical school curriculum. It can be done during earlier clinical pathology sessions, during clerkships, as part of grand rounds, and in continuing education.

7 Current Public Policies

> Health Care—a most fundamental and personal need—is being
> examined in a new light.
> —National Commission on the Cost of Medical Care, 1977

During the 1970s, the spiraling cost of medical care became a
primary concern for industrialized nations. The concern was particularly manifest in the United States, which, for historical reasons, had
not yet had to deal with scarcity and accountability. Expenditures on
health care have risen dramatically, and health-care services account for
a continually growing portion (now 10 percent) of the gross national
product.

> Physicians play a major role in determining the Nation's health care
> costs, and studies have shown that increased emphasis on training
> them in cost containment techniques can produce lower costs.
> GAO's review showed that, although progress is being made—
> primarily by medical schools, residency programs, and professional
> groups—to increase emphasis on such training, more needs to be
> done by both the medical profession and the Federal Government
> to foster the teaching of cost-effective medicine (GAO Report,
> 1982).

Since most educational programs in cost containment have a
particular, clinical orientation, they often do not address problems of
the health system. The AMA-sponsored study of cost containment
identified some of the more general problems that physicians should be
aware of in relation to health-care costs. A teaching strategy was
developed at the Medical College of Ohio, Toledo, in 1979 in which the
teaching of national issues of health economics was integrated into the
regular clinical clerkship curriculum.

104

DESCRIPTION OF CURRICULUM

The curriculum was integrated into the clinical clerkship in pediatrics. Using lecture and discussion, instructors presented the major national issues of the day and asked the students to relate the issues discussed to their experiences during their clerkship. No extra research assignments were given that would add weight to the students' workloads, and only a short paper was required for the final seminar. The curriculum was designed to deal with three pragmatic concerns: lack of teaching time, the necessity for curricular adaptability, and the need to minimize demand on students' time. Three and one-half hours of teaching time was involved.

Program Outline

Students first attended a one-hour introductory lecture in which a brief overview of health economics and the relationship of the physician to the health-care system was explained (Figure 7.1). During this lecture, students also were given background information on health-care inflation and the effect of specialization on health-care costs.

Two well-publicized events concerning health-care costs became the focus of the curriculum: a proposal from the Carter Administration for a nine percent ceiling on increases in hospital charges, and the release of a document by the American Medical Association (AMA, 1977), the Report of the National Commission on the Cost of Medical Care. The proposal and the report were outlined during the introductory lecture. The AMA National Commission Report contained 48 recommendations on how health-care costs could be brought under control. Each student was asked to read the Summary Report and write a two or three page discussion of two out of ten selected recommendations. They were asked to consider the recommendations in the light of the medical practices they were to witness during their forthcoming clinical clerkship in the hospital. Students were asked to discuss in their papers whether the recommendations were applicable to their clinical settings and would make practice more efficient while maintaining the best medical care for patients. They were also expected to present arguments, developed from their experiences, about whether or not they supported the recommendations.

During the third week of their pediatric clerkship, each group of 20 students participated in a two and one-half hour seminar and workshop. During the first hour, students discussed their findings and

FIGURE 7.1. Cost awareness in medical decision making I.

In preparation for the Cost Awareness Seminar, each student is required to answer the following two questions based upon the readings provided (Fineberg, H.V., and Hiatt, H.H.: "Evaluation of medical practices," N. Eng. J. Med. 301:1086 [1979]; Maloney, T.W., and Rogers, D.E.: "Medical technology—a different view of the contentious debate over cost," N. Eng. J. Med. 301:1413 [1979]) and upon his or her experiences during the Pediatric Clerkship. Each answer should be about one typed, double-spaced page.

1. Cite two examples of diagnostic approaches or therapies from your patient cases which used technologies recently (within 10 years) introduced into medical practice, discuss the benefits and costs (both money and complications), and give one example of how problems of cost-benefit may be resolved.

2. How can physicians' practices and decisions be refined and influenced to maintain quality but control cost? Cite two examples of how the management of your patients might have been modified to result in a less costly but equally effective outcome, and how limitations on availability of technology, as described in the strategies of Maloney and Rogers, might have affected (for better or worse) the care, outcome, and cost of your patients' management.

---

their views on the recommendations of the National Commission on the Cost of Medical Care. They were also asked to comment on the Carter Administration's proposals for a nine percent ceiling on increases in hospital charges and its possible effects on medical practice. Today, the same questions are being asked about diagnosis-related-groups (DRGs) reimbursement, which essentially places a ceiling on the reimbursement a hospital will receive for each Medicare patient.

Role Playing

During the second hour and 15 minutes of the seminar, a role-play session was enacted (Fig. 7.2). Each of 10 students in a given group was assigned a role. Students received cards on which their characters were described. Characters included were:

> chief of staff
> hospital administrator
> director of nursing services
> chief of laboratory services
> chairman of radiology
> chairman of medicine
> chairman of surgery
> chairman of pediatrics
> consumer advocate
> PSRO representative

The simulated hospital setting in which these characters were placed was a teaching, not-for-profit, community hospital of moderate size (500 beds), affiliated with a medical school. Occupancy rate for the hospital was 91 percent annually, with occupancy of the pediatrics unit at 96 percent. During the previous year, the hospital had made a request to expand to 650 beds, but the local planning agency had refused the request, citing under-utilization of other community hospitals as the reason for the denial.

Other factors that the students were to consider were that inflation was running at 10 percent per year, and hospital *costs* were increasing at 15 percent per year. The government had established a 9 percent ceiling for hospital charge increases.

Several problems were defined and each group of 10 students was assigned one of the following problems:

> Develop a hospital strategy to contain costs within the 9 percent ceiling.

> Because of the high occupancy rate, consider a plan to monitor and limit lengths of stay, provide preadmission certification, promote preadmission testing, and encourage an early discharge— home nursing program.

> Develop a strategy to increase physicians' awareness of the costs of the services they order.

> Justify a request by the Department of Radiology for the purchase of a CT scanner.

The chief of staff in each group chaired the sessions, and one participant was designated as the recorder. Each group was required to provide a written outline of its plan at the end of the session.

FIGURE 7.2. Cost awareness in medical decision making II.

ROLE-PLAY WORKSHOP

Objectives:

1. Gain understanding of group dynamics in medical decision making in the hospital organization setting.

2. Gain understanding of personal, technical, economic, and political factors involved in setting priorities for hospitals.

3. Utilize information gained from readings in a problem-solving situation.

Setting:

A 600 bed community hospital with a 45 bed pediatric service, including a six bed ICU, and a neonatal service with 30 bassinets and a 15 isolette intensive care (level three regional center) unit. The outpatient department has 12,000 visits per year in general pediatrics and subspecialties. Emergency room visits for children are 10,000 per year. The pediatric service averages 2/3 "private" patients and 1/3 "service."

The outpatient department services primarily an indigent (88 percent) population for general pediatrics and a referral population for cardiology, pulmonary medicine, neurology, and pediatric surgery.

In the community of 75,000 people, there are two other major hospitals, three neighborhood health centers run by the health department, 16 private pediatricians, and 20 family practitioners. The regional area served has 140,000 people. The two other hospitals have 60 pediatric beds and 24 nursery bassinets; one hospital has an outpatient department seeing 16,000 children per year and specialty services for pediatric endocrinology, nephrology, and gastroenterology.

Your hospital and another in town are affiliated with a medical school located 20 miles away. There are 15 pediatric residents (6 PL 1, 5 PL 2, and 4 PL 3) distributed between the two hospitals; 2 PL 1, 3 PL 2, and 4 PL 3 positions are currently unfilled. Six medical students are assigned to your pediatric service each month.

Occupancy rate for the pediatric ward runs 88 percent.

Roles:

1. Hospital Administrator—B.A. in hotel management, M.B.A. in hospital administration.

2. Director of Nursing Service—in position 14 years, traditional, "old-fashioned."

3. Director of Laboratory Services—a prominent pathologist; innovative, efficient.

4. Chief of Staff—a prominent surgeon, well respected; gentle and kind.

5. Chief of Pediatrics—an excellent clinician and teacher, liked by all; keen sense of humor.

6. Chief of Surgery—conservative, no-nonsense; "does not suffer fools in silence."

7. Chief of Medicine—quiet, well respected; hypertension expert.

8. Chief of Radiology—heads large consultant group.

9. Consumer Representative—a prominent businessman.

10. Health Planning Agency Representative—M.P.H. in medical care organization.

The preceptor will serve as observer, evaluator, and technical resource for demographic, economic, and legal information.

The Chief of Staff will chair and coordinate the meeting. Each member will introduce him/herself with a brief description of the role and background. The designated presenter will present the problem and its justification within ten minutes; he/she may call upon the preceptor for technical assistance. Committee members may then have three minutes for response and 30 minutes for general discussion. After a ten minute break, students, out of role, will have three minutes each to summarize the role-play session.

Problems:

1. The Radiology Department requests the purchase of a C.T. scanner with capability of body as well as brain scanning. The request is supported by the neurology staff and Department of Surgery. The H.P.A. notes that the medical school (20 miles away) has a C.T. scanner. None of the other hospitals in town has a C.T. scanner.

FIGURE 7.2. (*continued*)

2. The hospital has a 9 percent ceiling on increased expenditures. The Department of Pediatrics requests a renovation and expansion of the outpatient area, which is 20 years old. The H.P.A. supports the need based on increasing patient volume, inefficient layout of the present clinics, and the competition for space among the general pediatrics service and the subspecialty services. Similar problems exist for Internal Medicine and Surgery. The expenditure would create a 3 percent increase if only Pediatrics were renovated and an 8 percent increase if Pediatrics, Medicine, and Surgery were renovated.

3. In order to reduce costs, the hospital has limited the hiring of new personnel to a 2 percent increase of the current personnel budget. The Pediatrics Department has determined a need for 5 new nurses on the Pediatric Ward.

Problems are generally chosen from current events at the associated hospitals to lend a sense of immediacy and relevancy.

During the role-play sessions, the students became aware of some of the important factors involved in making decisions when competing interests, economic constraints, and different priorities were involved. The students were remarkable in their abilities to play their roles. Each workshop was unpredictable, but each group was consistently well-managed and efficient. The role-play sessions were, by agreement of both faculty and students, one of the most effective methods for teaching cost-containment and cost-awareness. Because of their familiarity with the issues from the report of the task force, the students were able to provide reasonable and stimulating arguments both for and against the implementation of the programs presented to them. The interchange among the students provided a realistic forum for the discussion of health-resources allocation and cost containment.

Faculty members served as observers and resource persons for specific technical or demographic information during the role-play sessions. For each problem presented, two students served as advocates and the rest of the group served as discussants or opponents to the proposal. It was frequently necessary to arrange a compromise among competing interests in order to solve the problem.

The advocates of the proposal were allowed ten minutes for their presentation, and each member of the group was allowed five minutes to respond before general discussion ensued. The moderator kept track of time and terminated general discussion 15 minutes before the end of the workshop session before taking final proposals and amendments. A faculty critique followed before the session was adjourned.

RESOURCE RECOMMENDATIONS FOR THIS CURRICULUM

1. Faculty

   a. One member with expertise in health economics to plan and coordinate seminars.
   b. Approval of a clinical department willing to allocate the limited time needed for such an activity.
   c. One member skilled in group-process techniques for the role-play session.
   d. A general discussion at the end of the role play involving as many of the appropriate hospital staff as possible to try addressing the same situation that the students did.
   e. As many clinical faculty as possible as discussants during the health-systems sessions to reinforce the importance of the non-clinical nature of the activity for students.

2. Materials

   a. Development of role-play materials, especially the details of the situation to be played out.
   b. Copies of the summary report of the National Commission on the Cost of Medical Care and a summary of the Diagnosis-Related-Groups Reimbursement regulations and methods.

3. Time

   a. Two seminar sessions, the first as introduction and the second reporting and role playing by students. The material should be distributed to students about five days before the first session to allow them to become familiar with some of it but not forget it before the seminar.

b. Seminars should be no longer than two weeks apart to avoid unnecessary repetition for some students.

c. Other faculty and administrative time would be needed for the appropriate segments.

4. Number of Students and Space

a. The number of students should be small enough for all to participate actively in the role play unless it is structured so that two student groups role play in different rooms and come together again to discuss their conclusions.

b. One or two seminar rooms should be sufficient.

5. Evaluation

a. For such a short curriculum, evaluation would have to be of the formative type, involving the primary faculty's questioning of other faculty to see whether students were asking certain questions of a systemic nature.

b. Again, to the extent that other faculty and administrators had been involved in the sessions, reinforcement and process evaluation of students could be more effective.

6. Locus in Curriculum

The program could be done equally easily in the basic or clinical curriculum segments. Reinforcement and bridging the gap between the health-system issues raised and the clinical practice would be important and a long-term process; therefore clinical segments would be preferable.

CONCLUSIONS

Despite the limitations of such a short health economics curriculum, students felt that these issues were important. Students became more aware of their role as physicians in cost-containment efforts and of the impact that regulatory efforts might have on their medical practices. They now have had experience in discussing the current national issues in health economics and were able to participate in a simulated decision-making process that involved the allocation of resources. The students came to understand that the problem of cost containment is one to be shared by the medical profession both individually and collectively, and by hospitals, the community, and the government. Finally, these medical students became aware that high cost is not necessarily synonymous with good medicine and that quality care can be cost effective.

Students' Comments on the Current Policies Seminars

Although the curriculum dealing with the AMA's cost commission and the role play was created in response to a shift in curricula (the college went from a 3-year to a 4-year program, and the mandatory community medicine clerkship was eliminated), it generated a good deal of reaction. Some of the students' observations on such controversial topics may provide some readers with useful insights into students' perspectives. They are presented here with that in mind.

Ten of the 48 recommendations issued by the National Commission on the Cost of Medical Care were used. The recommendations chosen were thought to represent the issues that would be of most immediate concern to the medical students when they entered their own practices. Another reason why these particular recommendations were chosen was that examples of how they could be applied were most likely to be found in the students' clinical experiences.

The ten recommendations selected for critique by students were:

Recommendation 14: Incentives to provide appropriate care
Recommendation 22: Placement review criteria
Recommendation 23: Regional centers
Recommendation 26: Diagnostic findings
Recommendation 27: Second opinions prior to surgery
Recommendation 30: Defensive medicine
Recommendation 38: Curricula on economics of health care
Recommendation 39: Price consciousness in the hospital setting
Recommendation 46: Health and patient education
Recommendation 48: Healthful lifestyles

Each student was assigned to offer a critique on two of these recommendations. Following is a review of the students' critiques of the assigned recommendations. Their views and the ways in which they were able to relate the issues involved in the recommendations to experiences they had on the wards are the best examples of how cost-containment training can be successfully integrated into any medical school curriculum.

Recommendation 14: Incentives to Provide Appropriate Care

A. On the basis of peer review criteria and findings, the medical profession, working through specialty societies and others, should develop and disseminate guidelines for appropriate care based on criteria of medical necessity, quality, and cost benefit. These criteria should be sufficiently detailed and explicit so as to identify departures from them and allow independent consideration of the medical appropriateness of such departures.

B. The medical profession, working with third-party payers, should explore ways to put providers at risk for at least part of the inappropriate care resulting from provider utilization decisions as indicated by unacceptable departures from the established guidelines relevant in a particular instance. Neither the patient nor third-party payer should bear the costs of decisions which result in inappropriate care.*

Student responses to this recommendation were almost universally negative. Most were disturbed by the word "guidelines." They thought that these might limit physicians' ability to use their professional judgment to treat the same disease in different ways depending on particular cases and conditions. One student said that certain guidelines in the treatment of specific diseases had already been established within the profession. He also noted that physicians are taught in medical school to treat each case individually because diseases can be unpredictable. He also pointed out:

Physicians are taught not only on an academic level but also on an intuitive level to diagnose, treat, and follow up disease. A test

*National Commission on the Cost of Medical Care: Summary Report. Chicago: AMA, December 1977. All further citations of recommendations are taken from this report.

ordered by a doctor on an intuitive basis may at times prove to be inappropriate, but may, in some cases, save an individual's life by providing the missing link in a complicated diagnosis.

In general, the students felt that physicians should be held responsible professionally for their performance and for the outcomes of their treatments rather than for their differences in approach and differences in the cost of treatments.

The students mentioned that the development of guidelines would simply add to the amount of bureaucratic paperwork that has already indirectly increased the cost of health care. Such "housekeeping" might become even less cost effective than the current system. Also, implementation of such guidelines would require the employment of more bureaucrats and would, again, add to the cost of care.

Some students pointed out that physicians would be put in a double-bind situation if guidelines were established. One student said that physicians would have to practice "reverse defensive medicine." Another student defines the problem in this way:

> Such a structure of making certain tests or procedures mandatory and others taboo would place physicians in the double bind of providing quality health care wedged between fears of malpractice for not investigating every possibility and being held primarily responsible for tests or procedures which ultimately turn out—retrospectively—to be unnecessary.

Many of the students did feel that physicians needed to "clean up their acts" and that, in many cases, physicians do need to become more cost conscious. Some students gave examples from their clinical experience of inappropriate use of tests. In one case, a student witnessed inappropriate use of tests to diagnose. An infant who had diarrhea was referred to the pediatric gastroenterologist on staff who proceeded to order a large number of laboratory tests aimed at finding an etiologic cause for the diarrhea, which was thought to involve the GI tract. It just so happened that a medical student and another attending physician examined the child's ears. It was discovered that the patient was suffering from otitis media. The tympanic membrane was the primary source of infection, and the infection was the sole cause of the diarrhea. The student commented that "a large amount of expense could have been saved had the attending physician and other medical staff been more aware that otitis media can often cause infant diarrhea."

Although most of the students recognized the problem of inappropriate use, none of them agreed with the solutions proposed in Recommendation 14. Students offered suggestions for a more "reasonable approach" to a cost-conscious policy. Some favored a more thorough peer-review system that includes making physicians aware of costs. One student thought that physicians could be made aware of costs if hospitals and laboratories were required to print the costs of procedures and studies on the report sheets that go to physicians. Students, in general, thought that neither the federal government nor anyone outside the medical profession could draw up appropriate guidelines that would ensure quality care.

Recommendation 22: Placement Review Criteria

Develop consensus criteria for the placement of expensive facilities and capital equipment, such as computed tomography (CT) scanners and open-heart surgery units, for use by state and local health-planning agencies in making placement decisions of this type. The criteria should be developed at the national level with the cooperation of expert health professionals, including providers and government, and should be flexible enough to meet specific needs of individual states and localities. The criteria should take into account factors such as medical need, operating as well as capital costs, and other expected benefits and costs of the specific technology. States might be given the option of exceeding the national criteria within established limits.

Most of the students thought that the concept of regional centers for high technology care and consolidation of expensive equipment and facilities was an acceptable and cost-effective solution to the problem of scarce resources and expensive technology.

However, several students mentioned problems that they had experienced or could anticipate in transporting patients to regional centers. One student found that transporting a patient who needed a heart scan was very awkward and inconvenient. The patient could not be transferred across town for the diagnostic test at the time he needed it most, and he could not be transported during the early phase of his hospital stay because the stress would have exacerbated his illness. The student remarked: "I cannot judge the economic advantage in centralizing facilities, but I can appreciate that such centralization very well could make facilities difficult or impossible to use." Another student said that in many cases it is expensive and traumatic for the patient to be transported from one facility to another. One student mentioned that even when transportation is available, some regional centers are now so crowded that it is difficult for patients to be admitted when they are in critical need of care at such facilities.

Some students felt that development of placement criteria for facilities and equipment at the national level with the cooperation of health professionals was an excellent idea. However, one student thought that the federal government should be kept as far away from these efforts as possible. This student remarked that the federal government would be unable to administer services well and that local regions should develop criteria and programs according to their own needs.

Another problem anticipated by the students was that hospitals would be reluctant either to give up existing services or to cancel plans for proposed services or equipment. As one student explains:

> Every hospital has a certain pride in supplying all "essential" services and some "nonessential" services. It will be very difficult to tell a hospital that it cannot have a CT scanner when every neurologist wants to use one. The hospital would lose its neurology service and the income from it.

Another student offered a three-point plan for determining how facilities and equipment should be allocated:

1. We should determine by retrospective and prospective studies how many facilities are needed, the type of patient who is going to need them, and the locations in which the greatest need and the largest number of patients are found.

2. We should try to meet the demands of the patients by putting these facilities in the optimum area for their convenience. Flexibility is important in this kind of project.

3. We should reduce the amount of jealousy, excessive pride, and politics that exists among professionals so that cooperation can be achieved in this endeavor.

Recommendation 23: Regional Centers

Where cost-saving opportunities exist, regional centers should be established for high-cost specialized technologies. The number of such opportunities may be limited. Separate planning systems which would fragment and overlap with CON (certificate of need) review should not be allowed to proliferate.

Capital expenditure restrictions are another method that could be employed to control resources. Under the proposed Hospital Cost Containment Act of 1977, each year the Department of Health Education and Welfare would limit total national hospital capital expenditures for resource development and/or renewal. Each state would be allocated a share of the total, based largely on the state's population. Planning agencies, using the CON mechanism, would determine how their state's share would be spent.

It is argued that the advantage of this approach, in contrast to other possible financing restrictions, is that it would effectively put a lid on capital spending while maintaining flexibility in terms of specific investment choices. Furthermore, it is argued that a capital expenditure limit might strengthen CON agencies in their decision-making roles by increasing their resistance to political pressure.

The proponents of capital expenditure limits have, however, failed to develop the valid methodology or reliable process to determine the appropriate level and distribution of capital expenditures. Moreover, the practical difficulties of determining the appropriate level of the limit make it very likely that, if enacted, its impact would be arbitrary and uneven.

The students' responses to this recommendation were favorable, and they were able to relate the recommendation to their experiences during their clerkships. Many of the students mentioned the specialized Neonatal Intensive Care Nursery at Toledo Hospital and the Pediatric Intensive Care Unit at the Medical College of Ohio as examples of what they considered an excellent use of regional centralization of "high-cost specialized technologies." One student said that such a highly-organized system is able to provide the most specialized care to the greatest number of patients in the most efficient and cost-effective manner. He also pointed out that "as personnel costs have been cited as the single most important factor in spiraling medical costs, the concentration of highly-trained personnel into regional centers seems to be a most cost-effective course."

One major problem that the students pointed out with regard to regionalization was who would make the decisions about where regional, special-care centers would be located. Several mentioned that increasing the bureaucracy in order to implement Recommendation 23 might increase costs. However, another student felt that only forceful directives from a powerful planning agency relatively free of political pressure will accomplish anything in the way of capital expenditure limitations. This planning agency should be nationwide, dividing the entire country into regional districts in which one institution in each area would be delegated as the center in which high-cost specialized care would be done.

He further notes that proliferation of services and expansion is already "out of sight" and that present CON mechanisms crumble in the face of power and money. He cites as an example the case of *Tulsa v. Oral Roberts*, whereby Oral Roberts University was able to build a hospital in spite of the rejection of its CON by the local review agency.

Recommendation 26: Diagnostic Findings

Providers, working at the local level, should develop mechanisms for the sharing of diagnostic findings for a given patient in order to avoid duplication of expensive diagnostic tests and procedures.

The students found that informal mechanisms for sharing test results were already working in environments in which they did their clinical clerkships. Many expressed the opinion that these informal mechanisms were important and necessary tools for reducing the duplication of tests. For example, patients often are referred from one institution to another, and X rays and tests are sent with the patient. One student reported that, during his clerkship, he witnessed a high degree of cooperation among hospitals and physicians in exchanging records and diagnostic test results on an informal basis. One student mentioned that formal mechanisms for obtaining records require signatures, forms, and delays. Such delays can make information requested useless.

The students gave several examples of instances in which tests were unnecessarily duplicated. In cases where patients received care in more than one institution, the possibility of test duplication was high. In addition, when tests were done in a physician's office and the patient was then referred to the hospital, tests often were repeated unnecessarily. Duplicate testing often is done when patients who are examined in clinics or in the emergency department are admitted to the hospital.

Several suggestions were made for implementing a policy of test sharing. A more nearly complete standardization of diagnostic findings was needed. Also, a central data bank could be established that would allow any and all data on each patient to be readily retrieved. Another important suggestion was that physicians should fill out more detailed discharge summaries. The students thought that their recommendations would have three major results: they would reduce the problems and lag time of getting results on patients; increase the reliability of results; and maintain the confidentiality of the physician-patient relationship.

The students decided that there were difficulties in taking the recommendations too far. Sometimes a patient's condition changes from one testing time to another and, therefore, additional testing is required. The reliability and quality of individual laboratories would have to be standardized. Several students concluded that the best care results from frequent and effective communication among all parties involved in supplying medical care.

Recommendation 27: Second Opinions Prior to Surgery

> Third-party payers, working with providers, should undertake conscientious evaluation of the methodologies and the results of current experimentation with coverage of second opinions prior to elective surgery. The long-term results and general adaptability of such programs should be evaluated in terms of medical-care quality, cost effectiveness, the cost and quality of alternative care provided in place of surgery, and the long-range medical implications for the patients who did not have surgery.

The students were split in their opinions about this recommendation. Those who opposed mandatory second opinion programs thought that the practice would not be cost-effective in the long run. Many were concerned about who would bear the cost of these second opinions. Other students felt that the studies that have been done on the cost-effectiveness and health benefits of second opinions for surgery were insufficient, possibly biased, and did not study long-term effects.

One student who was opposed to the recommendation defined some of the problems that second opinions could cause. The trusting relationship between the physician and patient could be harmed if second opinions became mandatory, and many patients might become confused if confronted with several opinions. The medical profession might also suffer in the eyes of the public. Several students felt that mandatory second opinions were an insult to the intelligence and judgment of good physicians. These students maintained that most physicians practicing today are quite competent and are interested in providing the best possible care for their patients.

Some thought that mandatory second-opinion programs would be cost-effective and would improve the quality of care provided. The very existence of second-opinion programs would act as a brake to the recommendation of questionable or unnecessary surgery. Also, these programs would encourage surgeons to examine alternatives to surgery for each individual patient. Another student pointed out that second-opinion programs would provide an excellent peer-review mechanism.

Recommendation 30: Defensive Medicine

A. Providers and courts should utilize guidelines for appropriate care—based on consideration of quality, medical necessity, cost effectiveness, and allowing for the varying circumstances of individual cases—for guidance as to what constitutes acceptable levels of performance on the part of physicians and other providers.

B. The medical and legal professions, working together with third-party payers, should examine the feasibility and desirability of having the resolution of professional liability claims placed outside the traditional courtroom-jury setting.

Students objected to Part A of the recommendation because they felt that, instead of discouraging the practice of defensive medicine, it would, in fact, encourage such practice. Physicians would have to adhere strictly to pre-established guidelines instead of treating each case individually. This would increase the likelihood that unnecessary tests would be performed as a matter of routine, and alternative diagnoses might be overlooked.

On the other hand, several students thought that the kinds of guidelines mentioned in Part A might help to reduce the physician's need to practice defensive medicine and would, therefore, help to reduce patient-care costs. Some students thought that increased emphasis on primary care and the importance of physician-patient communications should be considered along with this recommendation. Many students felt that unnecessary, so-called "routine workups," could be eliminated in many cases.

Reactions to Part B of the recommendation were not as strong as reactions to Part A. Generally, the students believed that the custom of settling malpractice suits outside of the traditional courtroom setting was already the prevalent practice. However, most students were opposed to mandatory out-of-court settlement. They indicated that the American legal system has its strongest roots in the courtroom-jury ambience and removal of the option of a jury trial would tarnish the concept of justice. They also believed that third-party payers should not participate in decisions made concerning defensive medicine. Insurers have done nothing to lose either in occasional payments or in increased rates, and should simply accept decisions about medical care that are made by the medical and legal professions.

Recommendation 39: Price Consciousness in the Hospital Setting

> Physicians should be encouraged to enter or acknowledge the cost or charge for hospital-based services. The hospital setting provides an ongoing opportunity to reinforce the physician's price consciousness. The forms on which the physician orders services for his patients can be used to focus his attention on the cost of treatment alternatives.

Students were generally favorable toward the practice of educating physicians and other members of the health-care community about the cost of tests. One student said that the problem of costs for services has always been discussed during rounds in all of his clerkships. He added that he had learned a great deal from the literature and from discussions in medical school concerning the cost of services, admission, and procedures. He feels that this kind of teaching has had a major influence on his attitude concerning cost decisions. Others pointed out that individualized cost decisions are difficult to make because so many physicians are unaware of the cost of tests and procedures they order.

Most of the students felt that physicians needed to become more cost conscious. They wondered whether physicians who were aware of costs would order as many unnecessary tests. The students had several suggestions as to how physicians could become more aware of costs. Laboratory-test charges could be included on physician laboratory-test order forms or could be posted in clinical settings and other physician work areas. Several students suggested that it would be helpful if physicians were presented with a tally of costs of the hospital services that they ordered for each patient. Others recommended that students and residents be required to mark the cost of all the services and tests that they ordered on the medical record.

One student gave an example of one hospital's cost-awareness program. The cost of various tests, procedures, and pieces of equipment often was discussed during rounds. In addition, students and residents often were asked why tests were ordered. It was discovered during one session that two tests—electrolytes and BUNs—were being ordered much too frequently with little justification. Just the questioning of the appropriateness of the tests caused a noticeable decrease in the number of tests ordered. Another example of how cost awareness can result in savings was given by a student who said that he had seen many physicians order several laboratory tests separately (at $7 apiece) that were included in the SMA 12/60 test series ($15 for 12 tests). The fact is that, if any three of the 12 tests included in the AMA 12/60 series are ordered, all 12 tests can be done more economically and with less blood than if they are ordered separately.

Recommendation 46: Health and Patient Education

> Consumers and patients would be encouraged and assisted to become more active and knowledgeable participants in making health care utilization decisions by:
> A. Developing health and patient education programs that inform consumers and patients about the costs and benefits associated with potential and alternative courses of treatment, and
> B. Emphasizing self-help education programs directed at well and worried-well individuals and groups to provide consumers with the information necessary to make the initial decision as to whether there are other alternatives open to them, such as self-care, bed rest, or use of nonprescription drugs or first aid.

This recommendation, along with two others involving the subject of consumer and patient education, was developed because the commission believed that "educational programs are important in providing knowledge and assistance to consumers and patients if they are to make cost effective utilization decisions. Such educational endeavors thus become an integral part of any plan to contain health care costs."

All of the students were sympathetic to the principle of educating the public. Education provides patients with a sense of control over their illnesses and an understanding of their part in caring for themselves. An educated patient tends to view the physician as a friend and helper rather than a person who is just doing a job. Education is also an important factor in reducing costs because patients can make economic decisions about medical care that are based on knowledge rather than emotion.

However, the students cited certain problems. Some students said that patients whose bills are paid by third-party providers have little incentive to practice preventive medicine or to educate themselves about medical matters. They felt that many individuals knowingly live unhealthy lives, and then, when problems occur, put themselves in the hands of medical providers because the third-party payer will handle the bills. High costs and difficulties with implementing consumer education programs have also discouraged community organizations, hospitals, and physicians from pursuing such projects. Another problem mentioned was that often patients and consumers are given instructions, but, because of psychological and social difficulties, are unable to follow them.

Recommendation 48: Healthful Lifestyles

Consumers should be encouraged and assisted to learn healthful practices by:

A. Educating and motivating them to adopt more healthful lifestyles.

B. Exploring methods of utilizing public communication more effectively in health education efforts directed toward motivating consumers to adopt healthful lifestyles.

C. Encouraging them, in appropriate risk groups, to utilize professional preventive health-care services which would permit the early detection and treatment, or the prevention, of illness.

The students supported educational efforts not only as a means of helping diseased patients to help themselves but also as a practical means of implementing preventive medicine. They saw the mass media as a major weapon in the battle to educate the public. On this issue, they were even in favor of involvement by the federal government.

Two areas where the students thought that effective patient and consumer education could be encouraged were in obstetrics and pediatrics. Using experiences from their clerkships in these areas, they made a number of recommendations for physician involvement in educational efforts. Several students mentioned that parents are particularly receptive to information about how they can promote healthy lifestyle habits in their children. Physicians can, for example, counsel mothers to avoid overfeeding their babies in order to prevent future obesity.

Also, obstetricians can influence pregnant women by providing information about birth defects and other problems that might be prevented if healthful habits are practiced during pregnancy.

Some problems with consumer health education were discussed by the students. Several mentioned that many physicians practiced the very unhealthful habits that they preached against, thus appearing to be hypocritical to their patients. One student thought that health education was necessary and important, but that it would require a great expenditure of time and money to implement appropriate programs. Another student noted that it would take many years to obtain information about the long-term benefits of preventive education programs in regard to mortality, morbidity, and cost-effectiveness.

After they had presented their opinions and comments about the nine recommendations during the third week of the pediatrics clerkship, the students were asked to make one more short report. During the fourth week of the clerkship, all of the students were asked to comment on Recommendation 38, which deals with medical school curricula on health economics. The instructors felt that the students would be able to offer valuable insights into how health economics could be included in medical school course work.

Recommendation 38: Curricula on Economics of Health Care

A. Medical, dental, and osteopathic schools should develop curricula designed to expose students to the economics of the care they deliver, the nature of resource scarcity, and a variety of health care settings.

B. With the sponsorship of appropriate professional societies and with the use of a good textbook, the economics of health care should be incorporated in courses as a part of professional training The material should be mandatory and subject to examination.

All of the students agreed that the economics of health care should be taught and that it should be incorporated into the curriculum at all medical, dental, and osteopathic schools. They emphasized that such a curriculum should be worked into the entire medical school experience.

Several students commented on why health economics is so important. One student said: "A substantial part of the burden to contain the cost of medical care undoubtedly rests on physicians. Therefore, it is absolutely necessary for medical students, as future physicians, to learn the economics of health care and be constantly aware of its costs." The student reminds us that health-care cost problems will be with us for a long time. Another student enumerated the reasons why it is important to teach health economics in medical school:

1. Physicians are the principal decision makers, therefore, potentially, they have the most control of health-care costs.

2. The federal government will seek its own solutions unless physicians can demonstrate some competence in this area and show that their control measures will be effective.

3. Methods of health-care practice and delivery are learned in medical school and residencies, therefore, the most effective educational program would be presented in medical school.

A third student commented that health-economics curricula should teach students not only how much tests, treatments, and hospital services cost but also how all of these costs add up and how they affect the whole health-care system.

The students commented on the content of a medical-school health-economics curriculum. Such a program should include a description of the health-care delivery system, identification of the factors underlying the rising cost of health care, a review and evaluation of existing research on the causes of health-care cost inflation, an evaluation of suggested changes in the health-care delivery system that would affect health-care costs, and a study of cost-containment policies designed to reduce costs while, at the same time, providing high-quality care. In addition, the curriculum should include information on the role of third-party payers, such as insurance companies and the government; how Medicare and Medicaid operate, an explanation of the National Health Insurance controversy; how Professional Standards Review Organizations (PSROs) are organized; and what people and organizations are attempting to do in various communities to reduce health-care costs.

Some students suggested specific topics for training in health economics. One suggested that students learn how to operate a private medical practice in a cost-effective manner, how to minimize costs for inpatient care, and how to educate patients. Others suggested that students should be exposed to a greater variety of health care delivery systems rather than concentrating on the teaching hospital. Clerkships should be offered in private office practice and in outpatient clinics. Also, each specialty department (that is, surgery, obstetrics/gynecology, pediatrics, etc.) should devote some time to defining for students the specific problems in health-care costs that affect each particular specialty.

The students felt that the teaching methods employed in implementing a health-economics curriculum would be important to the effectiveness of such a course. One student commented that "early in the medical school career, a student isn't very interested in such mundane things as cost. It is necessary to find ways to introduce this topic in a manner that is interesting and not overpowering." Students generally supported the recommendation that a textbook should be used in the study of health economics, and that the course should include written examinations. Some commented that to ensure motivation and participation, students' work ought to be graded. Several students suggested that more time should be allotted for health economics. Another student said that as much as three hours per week for four weeks should be spent on the subject in addition to assignments during clerkships.

Informal discussion, integration into clinical case rounds and conferences, and the support of clinical faculty were mandatory for an effective curriculum, according to many of the students. Seminars and workshops alone were seen as ineffective settings for teaching cost issues.

REFERENCES

1. American Medical Association National Commission on the Cost of Medical Care, Vols. I, II, III, Chicago, AMA, 1977.
2. American Medical Association: National Commission on the Cost of Medical Care—Summary Report. Chicago, AMA, December 1977.
3. The U.S. General Accounting Office. Physician Cost-Containment Training Can Reduce Medical Costs, HRD-82-36 (February 4, 1982).

8   Continuing Medical Education
for Practicing Physicians

> ...that which we are, we are—
> One equal temper of heroic hearts
> Made weak by time and fate, but strong in will
> To strive, to seek, to find, and not to yield.
> —Tennyson

Over $500 million was spent directly on continuing medical education (CME) activities in the late 1970s and physicians forfeited an additional $1.4 billion by taking time off to attend CME events (Haynes et al., 1984). Many states incorporated CME requirements into their medical licensing and renewal, and formal CME activities have increased rapidly in the past few years.

Established medical education conferences and programs have become available for credit and many new programs have been organized in many communities to meet the increased demand. As availability and accessibility of programs increased, the quality of programs improved with better coordination of activities and development of specific learning objectives. Conferences are available, sponsored by hospitals, medical societies, and medical schools.

The lessons learned from experience with medical students were used to develop a program to present the issues of cost containment and the cost consequences of medical decision making to practicing physicians. Two principles established in the student curriculum guided the strategy:

1. The routine incorporation of the costs of medical tests, procedures, and treatments into appropriate clinical education programs was acceptable to program organizers and presenters,

128

and perceived as logical and reasonable by participating physician audiences.

2. If programs emphasized good medical practice, that is, quality of care and careful decision making, then they would demonstrate optimum cost benefits.

The Northwest Ohio Cost Awareness Project (NOCAP) was initiated in 1980 to demonstrate the facility of incorporating cost information into CME activities (Garg et al., 1984). The project was supported by a grant from the National Fund for Medical Education and was developed in cooperation with the Ohio State Medical Association and an advisory panel from Northwest Ohio hospitals and county medical societies. NOCAP integrated cost information into regular CME programs sponsored by the county medical societies and by the large teaching hospitals in the area. The program was initially intended to increase the awareness and involvement of physicians in hospital cost containment. However, because of the reluctance of hospital administrators to share information about their cost, policies, and quality assurance procedures, the project changed its focus to physican education about the cost of medical decision making.

Topics for presentation were selected by the director of medical education of each county medical society and were of general interest to the society members. Program development and faculty selection were coordinated with the Office of Continuing Medical Education at the Medical College of Ohio. Programs consisted of clinical case presentations, topical (specific problems or disorders) presentations, and discussions of general medical management problems.

The physician audiences felt that cost-awareness education was logical and informative. Incorporating cost factors into medical pro grams did not add significantly to their time commitment. Most physicians were enthusiastic about discussions of comparative costs, particularly of drugs. They felt that cost is as logical an outcome of care as is palliation and cure.

DESCRIPTION OF THE CURRICULUM

The office of the Director of Medical Education assists in the selection of topics and speakers. Each presenter is given detailed suggestions depending on the type of presentation to be given. Not all types of presentations, such as descriptive physiology, are applicable; but case reports, diagnosis and treatment for diseases, and clinical-pathological correlation lend themselves easily to cost comparison and discussion.

For case studies or simulations, the hospital and diagnostic costs can be presented in a number of ways. Suggestions given to presenters include:

1. Display hospital costs. For example,

a. Room Costs
   (1) Regular room   — $$
   (2) ICU/CCU   — $$

b. Diagnostic costs   Number of tests   — $$
   (1) Clinical Laboratory   —   "   "   "   —   "
   (2) Radiology   —   "   "   "   —   "
   (3) Special studies   —   "   "   "   —   "
   (4) Other studies   —   "   "   "   —   "

                  TOTAL   Number   — $$

2. Cost under each category can be discussed with examples of tests or procedures that may be of questionable utility for such a clinical case, and cost-effective decision making is emphasized.

3. Handout materials should include the costs of the hospital stay whether or not detailed discussion is planned.

4. Flow sheets containing the costs of tests are useful. For example,

Hospital Day and Test Result

Test	Cost	Day 1	Day 2	Day 3
Chest X ray	27.00			
CBC	8.50			
SMAC-12	12.50			
ABG	50.00			
U/A	9.50			

Daily Total

Cumulative Total

An effective method of increasing cost awareness is the presentation of a comparative list of similar therapies or drug costs. Figure 8.1 presents a flow diagram for the investigation of anemia which lists the costs of the tests ordered, and Table 8.1 gives a list of iron preparation with costs for comparison. Discussion included the drugs prescribed

FIGURE 8.1.   Investigation of anemia.

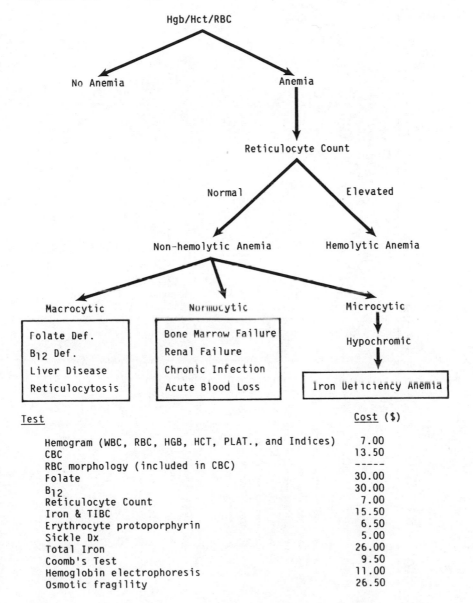

Test	Cost ($)
Hemogram (WBC, RBC, HGB, HCT, PLAT., and Indices)	7.00
CBC	13.50
RBC morphology (included in CBC)	-----
Folate	30.00
B$_{12}$	30.00
Reticulocyte Count	7.00
Iron & TIBC	15.50
Erythrocyte protoporphyrin	6.50
Sickle Dx	5.00
Total Iron	26.00
Coomb's Test	9.50
Hemoglobin electrophoresis	11.00
Osmotic fragility	26.50

TABLE 8.1. Cost of Some Iron Preparations*

Drug	Iron Content per Tablet, Capsule or Teaspoon	Approximate Cost per Gram of Iron
Ferrous sulfate, hydrated (20% iron)	60 mg	$ .15
average generic price (range: 7¢ to 23¢)		.16
Sugar-coated—average generic price (range: 8¢ to 39¢)		
Mol-Iron (Schering)	39 mg	.34
Timed-release—average generic price (range: 22¢ to $1)		.49
Feosol Spansule (SKF)	50 mg	1.32
Fero-Gradumet (Abbott)	105 mg	.62
Mol-Iron Chronosule (Schering)	78 mg	.65
Enteric-coated—average generic price (range: 5¢ to 39¢)	60 mg	.15
Ferrous sulfate, exsiccated (29% iron)		
Fer-In-Sol Capsules (Mead Johnson)	60 mg	.38
Feosol (SKF)	65 mg	.24
Ferrocholinate (12% iron)		
Chel-Iron (Kinney)	40 mg	.75
Ferrolip (Flint)	40 mg	.59
Ferroglycine sulfate complex (16% iron)		
Ferronord (Cooper)	40 mg	1.64
Vitamin-Mineral Products		
Adabee with Minerals (Robins)	15 mg	4.17
Chocks Plus Iron (Miles)	18 mg	1.64
Daylets Plus Iron (Abbott)	18 mg	2.65

Product	Iron	Cost*
Engran-HP (Squibb)	9 mg	5.58
Feminins (Mead Johnson)	18 mg	3.49
Femiron with Vitamins (JB Williams)	20 mg	1.52
Filibon (Lederle)	30 mg	1.88
Flintstones Plus Iron (Miles)	18 mg	1.64
Gerilets (Abbott)	27 mg	3.77
Geriplex (Parke, Davis)	6 mg	10.17
Geritol Junior Liquid (JB Williams)	16.5 mg	1.75
Geritol Liquid (JB Williams)	16.5 mg	2.24
Geritol Tablets (JB Williams)	50 mg	.93
Gevrabon (Lederle)	20 mg	12.62
Iberet (Abbott), timed-release	105 mg	1.24
Livitamin Capsules (Beecham)	33 mg	2.29
Myadec Capsules (Parke, Davis)	20 mg	3.94
Natabec (Parke, Davis)	30 mg	1.96
One-a-Day Plus Iron (Miles)	18 mg	1.69
Peritinic (Lederle)	100 mg	1.07
Poly-Vi-Sol with Iron (Mead Johnson)	12 mg	3.01
Stuart Prenatal Tablets (Stuart)	60 mg	.80
Therogran-M (Squibb)	12 mg	5.09
Unicap Therapeutic (Upjohn)	10 mg	8.07

*Cost of pharmacist, based on manufacturers' listings in Drug Topics Red Book, 1978, for purchase of 100 capsules or tablets or 16 ounces liquid where available; Average Wholesale Price used when given.

Reprinted with permission from: Medical Letter Vol. 21, 1979.

for the case, their costs, and alternatives that could have been used. Discussion could include the benefits (effectiveness, patient satisfaction and compliance, and side effects) of the drugs used or recommended in comparison with alternative therapy; it could also include judgmental conclusions regarding costs and benefits of the various choices.

For general medical-care management problems, it was suggested that the discussant define the problem and other related conditions and present management protocols. Alternative management methods could also be presented. The cost of treatment should be discussed using the management protocol and its alternatives, and conclusions should be stated regarding the benefits of the protocol. Such discussion could easily be combined with a case presentation.

RESOURCE RECOMMENDATIONS FOR COST-AWARENESS EDUCATION

1. Faculty

    a. Speakers should be chosen by the medical groups or hospital staffs through the Director of Medical Education.
    b. Faculty should be recognized for their expertise, credibility, and teaching ability, as well as for their interest in cost containment.
    c. Assistance from the Director of Medical Education or his staff may be necessary to provide cost information to the faculty.

2. Materials

    a. Hospital and laboratory charge information.
    b. Case records and billing information for case presentations.
    c. Library resources for cost-comparison information, such as, *The Medical Letter* and drug cost compendia.
    d. Cost (minimal) built into program cost where tuition or fee charged or figured into budget. Staff time should be no more than one hour for each presentation to collect cost information.

3. Time

    a. Preparation time should not add significantly to speakers' preparation time.

    b. Time for each program depends on the nature of the presentation.

    c. Cost-education programs should be presented regularly, if not integrated into all appropriate CME activities, so as to achieve optimum reinforcement of cost awareness.

4. Number of Participants and Space

    a. Depends on type of program.

    b. Not limited by scope and size.

A COMPREHENSIVE EFFORT

The recently enacted Medicare prospective payment legislation provides a renewed effort at containing rising hospital costs. Hospital administrators have now become intensely interested in programs to involve physicians in cost-containment strategies. The effectiveness of a program to stay within diagnosis related group guidelines will depend largely on physicians' cost conscious decision making (Enthoven, 1980).

Under these circumstances, educational programs based upon the utilization of ancillary services and ordering patterns will be needed very shortly. A comprehensive utilization review and education program has the advantages of being able to identify diagnoses with the widest variation in the use of ancillary services, to select topics for educational programs from these diagnoses, and to evaluate the impact of the educational program (McDonald et al., 1980; Schwartz and Hanson, 1982). The monitoring program generates data for comparative studies and identifies areas for improving efficiency.

As important as integrating cost awareness into CME is the selection of topics for discussion. One goal of continuing education is to encourage better utilization of resources. The need for containing costs within reimbursement guidelines is a major objective for practicing physicians and hospitals. At the same time, quality cannot be compromised. It is important to emphasize quality, cost-effective medical decision making.

Moloney and Rogers (1979) pointed out that high cost technology was not the major contributor to escalating costs. They demonstrated that greater savings were to be made by better selection of everyday tests and procedures. By identifying variations through review of ancillary services, cases and topics can be selected for educational programs that enhance efficient diagnostic management and treatment and minimize costs. Programs selected by utilization review can be mingled with programs on advances in medicine and those of selected interest to physicians.

Cost information should also be available to attending physicians and residents at the time tests are ordered or when results are posted (McDonald et al., 1980). Physicians and trainees thereby acquire a real "working" knowledge of the cost of their decisions. Training programs can no longer justify increased costs on teaching services for "education" or residents' inexperience. By knowing the cost of their decisions and by participating in CME programs that integrate awareness of costs, residents must appreciate the need for cost-conscious decision making at a time when they are forming their practice habits (Eisenberg and Williams, 1981; Eisenberg, 1982).

CONCLUSION

The inclusion of cost-awareness education in ongoing CME activities is logical, requires minimal preparation, and is acceptable to practicing physicians. Cost-of-care discussion blends easily into presentation of cases, clinical topics, and medical management. Although awareness of costs by itself may not have a direct impact on cost control, it provides physicians with a knowledge base upon which to participate in utilization review, priority setting, and allocation of resources (AMA Council on Medical Services, 1983). Awareness of cost alternatives provides one more factor in diagnostic and therapeutic decision making and emphasizes the need to be cost-effective (Weinstein and Stason, 1977).

Physicians are the "gatekeepers" of medical care, and their decisions influence almost 70 percent of hospital costs. Just as CME keeps them up to date in their practices, cost awareness helps them to put the advances in perspective and to be selective in their care. The benefits of careful decision making are quality medical care and optimal costs.

REFERENCES

1. Council on Medical Service, A.M.A. "Effects of Competition in Medicine." *JAMA* 249 (1983): 1864–1868.

2. Eisenberg, J.M., and Williams, S.V. "Cost Containment and Changing Physicians' Practice Behavior." *JAMA* 246 (1981): 2195–2201.

3. Eisenberg, J.M. "The Use of Ancillary Services: A Role for Utilization Review?" *Medical Care* 20 (1982): 849–861.

4. Enthoven, A.C. *Health Plan: The Only Practical Solution to the Soaring Cost of Medical Care.* Reading, Mass.: Addison-Wesley, 1980.

5. Garg, M.L., Kleinberg, W.M., Madigan, H.S., and Campbell, E.W., Jr. "The Northwest Ohio Cost Awareness Project." In *Persuading Physicians,* edited by Rubright, R. Rockville, Md.: Aspen, 1984.

6. Haynes, R.B., Davis, D.A., McKibbon, A., and Tugwell, P. "A Critical Appraisal of the Efficacy of Continuing Medical Education." *JAMA* 251 (1984): 61–64.

7. McDonald, C.J., Wilson, G.A., and McCabe, G.P. "Physician Response to Computer Reminders." *JAMA* 244 (1980): 1579–1581.

8. Moloney, T.W., and Rogers, D.E. "Medical Technology: A Different View of the Contentions Debate over Costs." *New Eng. J. Med.* 301 (1979): 1413–1418.

9. Schwartz, W.M., and Hanson, C.W. "Microcomputers and Computer-Based Instruction." *Journal of Medical Education* 57 (1982): 303–307.

10. Weinstein, M.C., and Stason, W.B. "Foundations of Cost-Effectiveness Analysis for Health and Medical Practices." *New Eng. J. Med.* 296 (1977): 716–721.

9   Epilogue and Prologue: Coming Full Circle

Our biggest problem in health care today boils down to one word: costs.

—Richard Schweiker, Secretary
U.S. Department of Health and Human Services, 1982

The growing concern about the escalating medical-care costs of the 1970s has continued into the 1980s, but the direction of response has shifted. In the 1970s we saw mandatory Professional Standards Review Organizations (PSROs) and Health Systems Agencies (HSAs) leading in cost containment, followed later by provider associations, such as the American Medical Association and the American Hospital Association, who sponsored a formal voluntary effort. Financial support for research and education in cost containment also came from the National Fund for Medical Education.

Unfortunately, evaluations of the PSRO program indicated that they cost the federal government more than they saved. The Certificate of Need approval mechanism used by HSAs to control capital expenditures also received mixed reviews and was often undermined by political considerations. In light of the increasing public frustration at the failure to control health-care costs, the Carter Administration proposed a cap on increases in hospital charges. The proposal was withdrawn only when a voluntary effort of provider associations was organized to control cost increases without government intervention. However, the voluntary effort also failed to control the costs of hospital care, with increases continuing at rates greater than the national inflation rate.

Some medical associations, professional societies, and medical schools began to develop their own cost-containment programs in the hopes of having some impact at the level of the individual practitioner

by attempting to change physician behavior. Some support was provided for such programs by the National Fund for Medical Education
over the past decade, including the Medical College of Ohio at Toledo
for many of the programs described in this volume.

However, two major obstacles persisted in the development of
medical-school education programs. One was the resistance of current
medical education leadership to the introduction of a new curriculum
for a problem that had been alien to medical education until recently.
Most of the leadership was trained at a time when technological and
scientific medicine was expanding rapidly, and public willingness to
support medical research and education seemed limitless. The optimis-
tic orientation was incompatible with the reality that resources are
limited, that cost containment must be allied with high-quality care,
and that more is not necessarily better.

The other obstacle was the lack of genuine support beyond a
handful of dedicated faculty members in just a few medical schools.
Some programs were designed for publicity rather than for serious
behavioral change. Moreover, many programs did not last beyond the
funding period, since a growing "critical mass" of clinical faculty was
not persuaded that such cost-effective clinical orientations need to be
emphasized to students.

Some hospitals and medical societies created cost-control programs consisting of "display" strategies as well as more sophisticated
and extensive chart review and cost-effective clinical decision-making
strategies. The "display" strategy simply is the posting of test costs or
regularly supplying physicians with copies of patients' bills. Such
strategies were never systematically evaluated and, lacking reinforcement, are unlikely to have a long-term impact. Some plans developed
computerized decision-making programs of clinical cases. The difficulty of such plans was the absence of broad-based clinical support and
reinforcement.

*One major lesson for educators becomes clear. Belief in cost containment
and cost-effective clinical decision making cannot be effectively taught
without an institutional policy, clinical support for the policies, and faculty
role-model behavior that explicitly indicates the importance of the program. It
is recommended that the continual involvement of as many faculty as possible
should be a key goal in development and planning of any cost-containment
program. Cost awareness and cost containment should be logical components
of medical care.*

The General Accounting Office of the Congress of the United
States has recently reviewed existing cost-containment programs, and

concluded that incentives should be given to medical schools to conduct such programs. However, the suggestion is focused on the teaching level and would require additional financial expenditures by the government or other sources. It is likely that the recommendation will be ignored, especially in an era of increasing resource limitation.

The prognosis for cost-containment programs in American medical schools is at best guarded. Some programs will go on because small numbers of faculty remain committed to the effort. Some have disappeared and others will continue to disappear. Over the next few years, any substantial effort in the area will come as an outgrowth of emerging prospective reimbursement policies. Medical care will be based increasingly on prospective (prearranged) payments, creating some incentives for hospitals to control costs. Some regions already have begun to develop programs in hospitals to change physicians' treatment behavior, particularly the excessive ordering of tests and procedures. When physicians are faced with *de facto* concurrent and prospective evaluation, their collective response will eventually trickle down to the medical-education level.

At the same time, the responsiveness of medical educators to the need for cost-containment education may be dramatically accelerated owing to prospective payment and the reimbursement provided to teaching hospitals. The initial Medicare regulations regarding prospective payment via DRGs permit the pass-through of medical education costs under the old cost-based system. Thus, teaching hospitals have some "breathing room" to contain some of those costs. At the same time, inexperienced residents who contribute to the hidden cost of medical education by ordering unnecessary tests for their own educational purposes, estimated at 10 percent of the tests in some studies, cannot be tolerated very long from the financial perspective of teaching hospitals. As such, the pressures on all hospitals to increase the efficiency of the clinical practices are even greater on teaching institutions. Both clinical faculty as role models and their students will have to become cost-effective practitioners, a situation dramatically different from educational practice to date. This of course raises new concerns about the control of clinical practice and quality of care, as well as the diffusion of clinical innovations.

The next educational efforts will have to address the problems of limited resources, efficiency in medical practice, and involvement in health services decisions. This new sense of urgency makes the programs described in this book, and programs yet to be developed, even more essential—both epilogue and prologue.

Selected Bibliography

Publications by the Authors

Garg, Mohan L., J.L. Mulligan, J.K. Skipper, and M.J. McNamara. "Teaching Students the Relationship between Quality and Cost of Medical Care." *Journal of Medical Education*, Vol. 50, 1975, pp. 1085–1091.

Garg, Mohan L., J.K. Skipper, M.J. McNamara, and J.L. Mulligan. "Primary Care Physicians and Profiles of Their Hospitalized Patients." *American Journal of Public Health*, Vol. 66, 1976, pp. 390–392.

Garg, Mohan L., W.A. Gliebe, and W.M. Kleinberg. "Quality in Medical Practice: A Student Program." *Journal of Medical Education*, Vol. 52, 1977, pp. 514–516.

Garg, Mohan L., W.A. Gliebe, and M. Elkhatib. "The Extent of Defensive Medicine: Some Empirical Evidence." *Journal of Legal Medicine*, Vol. 6(2), 1978, pp. 25–29.

Garg, Mohan L., D.Z. Louis, W.A. Gliebe, C.S. Spirka, J.K. Skipper, and R.R. Parekh. "Evaluating Inpatient Costs: The Staging Mechanism." *Medical Care*, Vol. 16(3), 1978, pp. 191–201.

Garg, Mohan L., Warren M. Kleinberg, and Werner A. Gliebe. "A Course on Costs and Quality." *Quality Review Bulletin*, Vol. 4(3), 1978, pp. 22–26.

Garg, Mohan L., W.A. Gliebe, and M. Elkhatib. "Medical Practices for Educational Purposes: The Internal Medicine Resident in a Teaching Hospital." *Hospitals JAMA*, Vol. 7(7), 1978, pp. 1–6.

Garg, Mohan L., J.L. Mulligan, W.A. Gliebe, and R.R. Parekh. "Physician Specialty, Quality and Cost of Inpatient Care." *Soc. Sci. and Med.*, Vol. 13C, 1979, pp. 188–190.

Garg, Mohan L., Werner A. Gliebe, and Warren M. Kleinberg. "Teaching Quality and Cost Through Student Peer Review of Diagnostic Tests." *Journal of Medical Education*, Vol. 54, November 1979, pp. 852–855.

Garg, Mohan L., Werner A. Gliebe, and Warren M. Kleinberg. "The Way We Teach Cost Containment." *Medical Teacher*, Vol. 2, No. 5, September/-October 1980, pp. 222–228.

Garg, Mohan L., Warren M. Kleinberg, and Werner A. Gliebe. "Cost Awareness in Continuing Medical Education: An Experiment." *Ohio State Medical Journal*, Vol. 76, November 1980, pp. 657–658.

Garg, Mohan L., Warren M. Kleinberg, Mounir B. Elkhatib, and Jack L. Mulligan. "Reimbursing for Residency Training: How Many Times?" *Medical Care*, Vol. 20, No. 7, July 1982, pp. 57–62.

Kleinberg, W., M. Garg, and W. Gliebe. "Cost Effective Medical Practices: A Curriculum at Medical College of Ohio," *Ohio State Medical Journal*, Vol. 75, May 1979, pp. 298–300.

Mulligan, Jack L., M.L. Garg, J.K. Skipper, and M.J. McNamara. "Quality Assurance in Undergraduate Medical Education at the Medical College of Ohio." *Journal of Medical Education* Vol. 51, 1976, pp. 378–385.

Skipper, James K., J.L. Mulligan, M.L. Garg, and M.J. McNamara. "Peer Group Review: An Educational Experience." *Ohio State Medical Journal*, Vol. 70, No. 2, 1974, pp. 488–490.

Skipper, James K., J.L. Mulligan, and M.L. Garg. "The Use of Peer Group Review in a Community Medicine Clerkship." *Journal of Medical Education*, Vol. 49, 1974, pp. 991–993.

Skipper, James K., G. Smith, J.L. Mulligan, and M.L. Garg. "Medical Students' Unfamiliarity with the Cost of Diagnostic Tests." *Journal of Medical Education*, Vol. 50, 1975, pp. 683–684.

Skipper, James K., G. Smith, J.L. Mulligan, and M.L. Garg. "Physicians' Knowledge of Costs: The Case of Diagnostic Tests." *Inquiry*, Vol. 13, 1976, pp. 194–198.

Other Related Publications

Berry, N.J. "PSRO Impact on Utilization: Forecast in a Cloudy Crystal Ball." *Hospitals*, 51, 1977, p. 57.

Brook, R.H., and K.N. Williams. "Effect of Medical Care Review on the Use of Injections: A Study of the New Mexico Experimental Medical Care Review Organization." *Ann. Intern. Med.*, 85, 1976, p. 509.

Buck., C.R., Jr., and K.L. White. "Peer Review: Impact of a System Based on Billing Claims." *New Eng. J. Med.*, 291, 1974, p. 877.

Burton, G.G., G.N. Glee, J.E. Hodgkin, and J.L. Dunham. "Respiratory Care Warrants Studies for Cost Effectiveness." *Hospitals* 49, 1975, p. 61.

Congressional Budget Office. *The Effect of PSRO's on Health Care Costs: Current Findings and Future Evaluations.*: Government Printing Office, 1979.

Dixon, R.H., and J. Laszlo. "Utilization of Clinical Chemistry Services by Medical Housestaff." *Arch. Intern. Med.* 134, 1974, p. 1064.

Eisenberg, J.M. "Educational Program to Modify Laboratory Use by Housestaff." *J. Med. Educ.* 52, 1977, p. 578.

Fineberg, H.V. "Clinical Chemistries: The High Cost of Low Cost Technologies." In Altman, S., and Blendon, R. (Eds.): *Medical Technology: The Culprit behind Health Care Costs?* Proceedings of the Sun Valley Forum on National Health. U.S. Dept. H.E.W., Pub. No. 79–3216, pp. 144–165.

Friedman, E. "Changing the Course of Things: Costs Enter Medical Education." *Hospitals*, 54, 1979, p. 82.

Galen, R.S. and S.R. Gambino. *Beyond Normality: The Predictive Value and Efficiency of Medical Diagnosis.* New York: John Wiley & Sons, 1975.

Galen, R.S. "Beyond Normality: An Update." In Benson, E.S. and M. Rubin (Eds.): *Logic and Economics of Clinical Laboratory Use.* New York: Elsevier/North Holland and Biomedical Press, 1978, p. 104.

Gorry, G.A., S.G. Pauker, and W.B. Schwartz. "The Diagnostic Importance of the Normal Finding." *New Eng. J. Med.* 298, 1978, p. 486.

Greenberg, D.S. "Cost-containment: Another Crusade Begins. *New Eng. J. Med.* 296, 1977, p. 699.

Greenland, P., A.I. Mushlin, and P.F. Griner. "Discrepancies between Knowledge and Use of Diagnostic Studies in Asymptomatic Patients." *J. Med. Educ.* 54, 1979, p. 863.

Griner, P.F. and medical housestaff, Strong Memorial Hospital. "Use of Laboratory Tests in a Teaching Hospital. Long-term Trends." *Ann. Intern. Med.* 75, 1971, p. 157.

Hardwick, D.F., P. Vertinsky, R.T. Barth, et al. "Clinical Styles and Motivation: A Study of Laboratory Test Use." *Medical Care* 13, 1975, p. 397.

Hudson, J.L., and J.D. Braslow. "Cost Containment Efforts in the United States Medical Schools." *J. Med. Educ.* 54, 1979, p. 835.

Kelly, S.P. "Physicians' Knowledge of Hospital Costs." *J. Fam. Pract.* 6, 1978, p. 171.

Kirkland, L.R. "The Physician and Cost Containment." *JAMA* 242, 1979, p. 1032.

Knapp, D.A., M.K. Speedie, and D.M. Yaeger. "Drug Prescribing and Its Relation to Length of Hospital Stay." *Inquiry* 17, 1980, p. 254.

Koran, L.M. "The Reliability of Clinical Methods, Data, and Judgment. Part 1." *New Eng. J. Med.* 293, 1975, p. 642.

Koran, L.M. "The Reliability of Clinical Methods, Data, and Judgment. Part 2." *New Eng. J. Med.* 293, 1975, p. 695.

Lawrence, R.S. "The Role of Physician Education in Cost Containment." *J. Med. Educ.* 54, 1979, p. 841.

Lewis, H.L. "Who Makes Decisions about New Technology in Hospitals." *Hospitals* 53, 1979, p. 114.

Lyle, C.B., R.F. Bianchi, J.H. Harris, et al. "Teaching Cost Containment to House Officers at Charlotte Memorial Hospital." *J. Med. Educ.* 54, 1979, p. 856.

Martin, A.R., M.A. Wolf, L.A. Thibodeau, et al. "A Trial of Two Strategies to Modify the Test Ordering Behavior of Medical Residents." *New Eng. J. Med.* 303, 1980, p. 1330.

McDermott, W. "Evaluating the Physician and His Technology." *Daedalus* 106, 1977, p. 135.

McNeil, B.J., E. Keeler, and S.J. Adelstein. "Primer on Certain Elements of Decision Making." *New Eng. J. Med.* 293, 1975, p. 211.

McNerney, W.J. "Control of Health Care Costs in the 1980's." *New Eng. J. Med.* 303, 1980, p. 1088.

Moore, S. "Cost Containment through Risk-sharing by Primary Care Physicians." *New Eng. J. Med.* 300, 1979, p. 1359.

Nagurney, J.T., R.L. Braham, and G.G. Reader. "Physician Awareness of Economic Factors in Clinical Decision Making." *Medical Care* 17, 1979, p. 727.

Pauker, S.G., and J.P. Kassirer. "Therapeutic Decision Making: A Cost Benefit Analysis." *New Eng. J. Med.* 293, 1975, p. 229.

Pineault, R. "The Effect of Medical Training Factors on Physician Utilization Behavior." *Medical Care* 15, 1977, p. 51.

Pozen, M.W., and H. Gloger. "The Impact on House Officers of Educational and Administrative Interventions in an Outpatient Department." *Soc. Sci. Med.* 10, 1976, p. 491.

Relman, A.S. "The New Medical Industrial Complex." *New Eng. J. Med.* 303, 1980, p. 963.

Rhyne, R.L., and S.H. Gelbach. "Effects of an Educational Feedback Strategy on Physician Utilization of Thoid Function Panels." *J. Fam. Pract.* 8, 1979, p. 1003.

Rogers, D.E. "On Technologic Restraint." *Arch. Intern. Med.* 135, 1975, p. 1393.

Roth, J.A. "The Necessity and Control of Hospitalization." *Soc. Sci. Med.* 6, 1972, p. 425.

Sackett, D.L. "Laboratory Screening: A Critique." *Fed. Proc.* 34, 1975, p. 2157

Schroeder, S.A., and D.S. O'Leary. "Differences in Laboratory Use and Length of Stay between University and Community Hospitals." *J. Med. Educ.* 52, 1977, p. 418.

Schroeder, S.A., K.I. Marton, and B.L. Strom. "Frequency and Morbidity of Invasive Procedures. Report of a Pilot Study from Two Teaching Hospitals." *Arch. Intern. Med.* 13, 1978, p. 1809.

Schroeder, S.A., and J.A. Showstack. "Financial Incentives to Perform Medical Procedures and Laboratory Tests: Illustrative Models of Office Practice." *Medical Care* 16, 1978, p. 289.

Schroeder, S.A. "Variations in Physician Practice Patterns: A Review of Medical Cost Implications." In Carels, E.J., D. Neuhauser, and W.B. Stason. *The Physician and Cost Control.* Cambridge, Mass.: O. B. & H. Pubs., Inc., 1980, pp. 23–50.

Schroeder, S.A., K. Kenders, J.K. Cooper, et al. "Use of Laboratory Tests and Pharmaceuticals: Variation among Physicians and Effect of Cost Audit on Subsequent Use." *JAMA* 225, 1973, p. 969.

Schwartz, W.B., G.A. Gorry, J.P. Kassirer, and A. Essig. "Decision Analysis and Clinical Judgment." *Amer. J. Med.* 55, 1973, p. 459.

Scitovsky, A. "Changes in the Use of Ancillary Services for 'Common' Illness." In Altman, S.H. and R. Blendon (Eds.): *Medical Technology: The Culprit behind Health Care Costs?* U.S. Dept. HEW, Pub. No. 79–3216, pp. 39–56.

Showstack, J.A., S.A. Schroeder, and H.R. Steinberg. "Evaluating the Costs and Benefits of a Diagnostic Technology: The Case of Upper Gastrointestinal Endoscopy." *Medical Care* Vol. 19, 1981, p. 49.

Smith, D.M., S.D. Roberts, and T.L. Gross. "Components of the Costs of Care for Medicine Patients at an Urban Care Center." *Clin. Res.* 27, 1979, p. 284A.

Tullis, J.L. "Are All These Lab Tests Really Worth It?" *Resident and Staff Physician*, Vol. 11, June 1973, p. 42.

Walker, K. "Commentary." In Benson, E.S., and M. Rubin (Eds.): *Logic and Economics of Clinical Laboratory Use.* New York: Elsevier/North Holland and Biomedical Press, 1978, p. 150.

Wennberg, J.E., L. Blowers, R. Parker, and A.J. Gittelsohn. "Changes in Tonsillectomy Rates Associated with Feedback and Review." *Pediat.* 59, 1977, p. 821.

Zeleznik, C., and J.S. Gonnella. "Jefferson Medical College Student Model Utilization Review Committee." *J. Med. Educ.* 54, 1979, p. 848.

Zieve, L. "Misinterpretation and Abuse of Laboratory Tests by Clinicians." *N.Y. Acad. Sci. Ann.* 134, 1966, p. 563.

Index